Installation Instructions

Windows

Step 1. Insert CD into your CD-ROM drive.

Step 2. After a few moments, the CD-ROM menu will automatically open.

Step 3. Select the item to install.

If the CD-ROM Menu does not automatically open, from the START Menu, select RUN and enter X:\SETUP.EXE (where "X" is the letter of your CD-ROM drive) and select OK.

Minimum System Requirements

PC

233 MHz processor
128 MB of RAM (256 MB of RAM recommended)
1024 x 768 resolution monitor
Windows 2000/XP/Vista
8x CD-ROM drive
150 MB of available hard disk space

MW006416512

LICENSE AGREEMENT

1. F. A. Davis ("FAD") grants the purchaser of *Student Resource Disk to Accompany NCLEX-PN Notes: Course Review and Exam Prep*, limited license for the program on the download CD-ROM ("Software"). FAD retains complete copyright to the Software and associated content.

2. Licensee has nonexclusive right to use this copy of the Software on one computer on one screen at one location. Any other use is forbidden.

3. Licensee may physically transfer the Software from one computer to another, provided that it is used on only one computer at any one time. Except for the initial loading of the Software on a hard disk or for archival or backup purposes, Licensee may not copy, electronically transfer, or otherwise distribute copies.

4. This License Agreement automatically terminates if Licensee fails to comply with any term of this Agreement.

5. SOFTWARE UPDATES. Updated versions of the Software may be created or issued by FAD from time to time. At its sole option, FAD may make such updates available to the Licensee or authorized transferees who have returned the registration card, paid the update fee, and returned the original CD-ROM to FAD.

LIMITED WARRANTY AND DISCLAIMER

FAD warrants that the CD-ROM on which the Software is furnished will be free from defects for sixty (60) days from the date of delivery to you by FAD or FAD's authorized representative or distributor. Your receipt shall be evidence of the date of delivery. The Software and accompanying materials are provided "as is" without warranty of any kind. The complete risk as to quality and performance of a nonwarranted program is with you.

FAD makes no warranty that the Software will meet your requirements or that Software operation will be uninterrupted or error free or that Software defects are correctable. No oral or written information or advice given by FAD, its dealers, distributors, agents or employees shall create warranty or in any way increase the scope of this limited warranty.

REMEDIES. FAD's entire liability and your exclusive remedy shall be limited to replacing the defective media if returned to FAD (at your expense) accompanied by dated proof of purchase satisfactory to FAD not later than one week after the end of the warranty period, provided you have first received a Return Authorization by calling or writing FAD in advance. The maximum liability of FAD and its licensors shall be the purchase price of the software. In no event shall FAD and its licensors be liable to you or any other person for any direct, indirect, incidental, consequential, special, exemplary, or punitive damages for tort, contract, strict liability, or other theory arising out of the use of, or inability to use, the software.

ENTIRE AGREEMENT. This Agreement contains the entire understanding of the parties hereto relating to the subject matter hereof and supersedes all prior representations or agreements.

GOVERNING LAW. This Agreement and Limited Warranty are governed by the laws of the Commonwealth of Pennsylvania. All warranty matters should be addressed to F.A. Davis Publishers, 1915 Arch Street, Philadelphia, PA 19103.

NCLEX–PN
Notes

Course Review and Exam Prep

Allison Hale,
MSN, BA, RN

Golden M. Tradewell,
PhD, RN

Purchase additional copies of this book at your
health science bookstore or directly from F.A. Davis
by shopping online at www.fadavis.com or by
calling 800-323-3555 (US) or 800-665-1148 (CAN)

A Davis's Notes Book

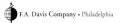
F.A. Davis Company • Philadelphia

F. A. Davis Company
1915 Arch Street
Philadelphia, PA 19103
www.fadavis.com

Printed in China by Imago

Last digit indicates print number: 10 9 8 7 6 5 4 3 2 1

Publisher, Nursing: Robert G. Martone
Senior Developmental Editor: William Welsh
Director of Content Development: Darlene D. Pedersen
Senior Project Editor: Padraic J. Maroney
Manager of Art & Design: Carolyn O'Brien

Consultants: Georgia Anderson, RN, MSN; Patrice P. Balkcom, RN, MSN; Patricia Beam, MSN, RN-BC; Eileen Beck, ADN, BSN; Marilyn S. Brady, PhD, RN; Beverly M. Brown, Ed.D, RN, MSN, ARPN/GCNS, BC; Diana Brumm; Renee T. Burwell, ASN, BSN, MSEd, EdD; Brigitte L. Casteel, RN, MSN; Pati L.H. Cox, RN, BSN, M.Ed.; Robin Culbertson, RN, MSN, EdS; Teresa Faust, RN, MSN; Joanne Folstad, BSN, Med(c); Brenda Walters Holloway, ARN-BC, FNP, DNSc; Maria E. Mackey, MSN, RN; Aimee W. McDonald, RN, MSN, ENP; Barbara McGraw, MSN, RN; CNE; Martha Olson, MSN, RN; Christine Ouellette, BSN, MSN, GNP; Cindy Lee Sherban, RN, BSCN; MAdEd; Martha M. Tingley, RN, MSN; Gerry Walker, MSN, RN; Kathy Wishon, RN; Bruce Wilson, PhD, RN, CNS, BC

As new scientific information becomes available through basic and clinical research, recom-mended treatments and drug therapies undergo changes. The author(s) and publisher have done everything possible to make this book accurate, up to date, and in accord with accepted stan-dards at the time of publication. The author(s), editors, and publisher are not responsible for errors or omissions or for consequences from application of the book, and make no warranty, expressed or implied, in regard to the contents of the book. Any practice described in this book should be applied by the reader in accordance with professional standards of care used in regard to the unique circumstances that may apply in each situation. The reader is advised always to check product information (package inserts) for changes and new information regarding dose and contraindications before administering any drug. Caution is especially urged when using new or infrequently ordered drugs.

Sticky Notes

✓ HIPAA Compliant
✓ OSHA Compliant

Look for our other Davis's Notes titles available now!

IV Therapy Notes: Nurse's Clinical Pocket Guide
ISBN-13: 978-0-8036-1288-4

LabNotes: Guide to Lab & Diagnostic Tests, 2nd edition
ISBN-13: 978-0-8036-2138-1

LPN Notes: Nurse's Clinical Pocket Guide, 2nd edition
ISBN-13: 978-0-8036-1767-4

MedSurg Notes: Nurse's Clinical Pocket Guide, 2nd edition
ISBN-13: 978-0-8036-1868-8

RNotes®: Nurse's Clinical Pocket Guide, 3rd Edition
ISBN-13: 978-0-8036-2313-2

PsychNotes: Clinical Pocket Guide, 2nd edition
ISBN-13: 978-0-8036-1853-4

For a complete list of Davis's Notes and other titles for health care providers, visit www.fadavis.com.

Preparing for The NCLEX-PN® Examination

Other than reviewing nursing content and practicing questions for the NCLEX-PN® Examination, the single <u>most important</u> thing that you can do to prepare for the exam is to print and review a copy of the NCLEX-PN® Test Plan from the following Web site:

- National Council of State Boards of Nursing (NCSBN). (2008). 2008 NCLEX-PN® Test Plan. Available at: https://www.ncsbn.org/ 2008_PN_Test_Plan_Web.pdf
- National Council of State Boards of Nursing (NCSBN). (2008). Resource Manual for International Nurses. Available at: https://www.ncsbn.org/ 08_Manual_for_International_nurses.pdf

- NCLEX-PN® measures the knowledge, skills, and abilities for entry-level practical/vocational nurses.
- Entry-level practical/vocational nurses must be able to meet the needs of patients who require the promotion, maintenance, or restoration of health under the direction of a qualified health professional.
- Integrated processes included within the client needs categories include clinical problem-solving process (nursing process), caring, communication/documentation, and teaching/learning.
- Practical/vocational nurses contribute to the interdisciplinary team in a variety of settings.
- The majority of test items are written at the application level or higher.

NCLEX-PN® Test Plan-Distribution of Content

Client Needs Categories	% of Items
Safe and Effective Care Environment	
• Coordination of Care	12–18
• Safety/Infection Control	8–14
Health Promotion and Maintenance	7–13
Psychosocial Integrity	8–14

Continued

Client Needs Categories	% of Items
Physiological Integrity	
• Basic Care/Comfort	11–17
• Pharmacological Therapies	9–15
• Reduction of Risk Potential	10–16
• Physiological Adaptation	11–17

Taking NCLEX-PN®

- NCLEX-PN® examination is administered using computer-assisted testing (CAT).
- Examination items are primarily multiple choice with four answer options.
- Alternate formats include multiple response, fill-in-the-blank, hot spot, drag and drop, and chart/exhibits.
- All item formats, including standard multiple choice, may have charts, tables, or graphic images.
- Candidates must answer a minimum of 85 questions and may answer a maximum of 205 during a 5-hour maximum testing period.
- Of these items, 25 are pilot test items that are not scored.
- To pass the exam, a candidate must **perform at or above** the passing standard.
- The candidate views the items one at a time on a computer screen. It is not possible to go back to a previous item once the candidate selects an answer and confirms the selected answer by pressing the <NEXT> button.
- Candidates must answer every item even if he or she is not sure of the correct answer because the computer will not allow the candidate to proceed to the next item without answering the item on the screen.
- If the candidate is unsure of the correct answer, he or she must make a "best guess" and move on to the next item.
- The best advice is (1) to maintain a reasonable pace, perhaps one item every minute or two, and (2) to carefully read and consider each item before answering. It is better to run out of time than to engage in rapid guessing.

Go to www.NCSBN.org to access an NCLEX® tutorial to practice multiple choice and alternate format items on the computer.

General Study Skills

- Ask yourself questions about the material that you have read.
- Form study groups.
- Make notes of key concepts or facts.
- Be interested in the material.
- Set specific goals.
- Establish a schedule for each day's studying and reviewing.
- Write summaries on what you read.
- Visualize the information you want to learn.
- Outline the key material that you just learned.
- Keep stress to a minimum.

Tips on Taking NCLEX-PN®

Multiple Choice Questions

- Use logic and common sense to figure out the correct response.
- Use cues in the question and options to help figure out the correct response.
- If a word in the question is identical, similar, paraphrased, or closely related to a word in the stem, then that option is most likely the correct answer.
- Try to figure out the meaning of unfamiliar words in the question.
- Read all options before selecting the one you think is correct.
- Eliminate the options that are obviously incorrect.
- Do not try to make an item any more difficult than it is. Do not "read into" the question.
- Relate each option to the question.
- Focus on key words in the question.
- Select the option that is most inclusive.
- Break down complex questions into smaller, more manageable sections.
- Make certain that the response you select is correct for each of the separate components.
- Try answering the question before you have read the options given.
- Concentrate on one item at a time.

- Focus on whether the question is asking for a positive or negative response:
  - A positive response question attempts to determine if you can understand, apply, or differentiate correct information.
  - A negative response question will have words in the question that are false, such as **except, contraindicated, unacceptable, least, avoid, violate, untrue, side effect, and exception**. Change a negative word to a positive word and then answer the question.
- Identify words that set a priority, such as the words **initial, main, primarily, initially, greatest, best, first, most, and priority**. If you are unable to identify a correct answer, eliminate the least desirable option and repeat again until left with a final option.
- If two options reflect extremes, such as hypo- vs. hyper-, increase vs. decrease, and brady- vs. tachy-, then identify what is associated with the opposite.
- Identify patient-centered options. Correct answers focus on feelings, choices, empowerment, and preferences.
- Eliminate options with "absolute" terms, such as **all, just, none, only, never, every, and always**. Options with absolute terms are generally incorrect.
- Eliminate options that deny a patient's feelings, give false reassurances, focus on the nurse, encourage cheerfulness, or change the subject.
- If three options to a question are similar in some way and one is different, the unique option often is the correct answer.
- If a question requires calculation, talk yourself through each step of the process.
- Use the steps of the nursing process. Remember that unless a life-threatening emergency exists, a nurse should always assess the situation first before taking action.
- Reword difficult questions.
- Look for the most common or typical response to the problem.
- Never leave an item unanswered.
- Use multiple test-taking tips to answer the question. Analyze the options for one or more test-taking tips.

Focus on what the question is asking and use the process of elimination to rule out incorrect options and to select the correct option. Use Maslow's Hierarchy of Needs as a guide to identify an intervention in relation to the question.

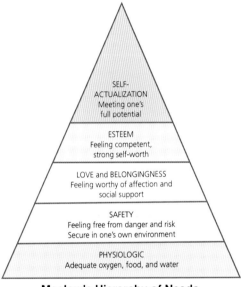

Maslow's Hierarchy of Needs

Tips for Answering Alternate Format Questions

Hot Spot Questions

"Hot spot" questions ask candidates to identify an area on a picture or graph by placing an "X" on the correct location.

The answer must mirror the correct answer <u>exactly</u> to receive credit.

Use the computer mouse and direct the cursor to the correct "spot" to answer the question.

When asked to identify an anatomical location, close your eyes, visualize the area, briefly recall the significant structures and functions, and then look at the picture.

When questions involve graphs or tables, first break them into segments for analysis and then review them as a whole.

Chart/Exhibit Questions

"Chart/exhibit" questions present candidates with a problem and require them to read the information in the chart/exhibit to answer the problem.

First, identify what the question is asking, then click each tab to collect data.

Compare and contrast the information collected in light of what the question is asking.

Recall information and compare it to the information in context of the situation presented in the question.

Drag and Drop Questions

"Drag and drop" questions require candidates to rank order, or prioritize, and move options to provide the correct answer.

The questions present a scenario or make a statement and then list a variety of actions or factors that must be placed in sequence or in order of priority. Choose the sequence that is identical to the correct response to receive credit.

Identify the action you believe should be first. Identify the action you believe to be last.

Evaluate the remaining two actions and make a final determination as to which one goes second.

Place the remaining action third.

Fill-in-the-Blank Questions

- "Fill-in-the-blank" questions require a mathematical computation, such as computing a drug dosage, calculating an intake and output, or determining the amount of IV solution to be infused.
- The recorded answer must be identical to the correct answer to receive credit. You do not have to type in the unit of measurement.
- Before attempting to answer the question, recall information related to the question, such as memorized equivalents or formulas to calculate IV drip rates. This taps your knowledge first and limits confusion.
- Type in the number(s) in a calculation item.

Multiple Response Questions

- "Multiple response" questions require candidates to select more than one correct option. They ask a question and then list several options; candidates must identify the options that are correct.
- Select all correct options to receive credit.
- Before looking at presented options, quickly recall information about the topic. This taps your knowledge first and limits confusion after looking at presented options.
- Compare your list to presented options; some of your recalled information should match. Then review the remaining presented options and determine if they are applicable.
- If you look at the presented options first, eliminate all incorrect options, then identify at least one or two you believe are correct.
- Finally, evaluate the remaining options and determine if they are correct or not.

Guidelines for International/English as Second Language (ESL) Student

Nurses from other countries who plan to work in the United States should have the following in order to become licensed in the United States:

- Comparable nursing education.
- English language proficiency to safely practice in the U.S. health-care environment.
- No current or previous disciplinary or criminal actions related to their current or previous license/registration to practice nursing.

- Successful completion of NCLEX-PN® licensing examination.
- No fraudulent or other illegally obtained documentation related to the verification of their required nurse credentials.

Research has identified several strategies that may help international/ESL students successfully pass the NCLEX-PN® exam. NCSBN (2008) has a Resource Manual for International Nurses.

- Language proficiency can be divided into two parts: linguistic competence and communicative competence.
- Linguistic competence uses grammatically correct phrases and sentences.
- Communicative competence receives, processes, and provides information accurately, thus increasing social acceptability and appropriateness.
- Language skills are a key factor in passing the NCLEX-PN® exam.
- Language proficiency is necessary for international/ESL students to become successful in the workplace.
- Use videos for learning, review content learned in the nursing program, participate in study groups, ask questions, and attend workshops.
- Learning activities, which include stimulation of more than one sense (i.e., not only audio) contribute to learning.
- International/ESL students should repeat questions to English-speaking peers to enhance verbal skills.
- Using medical terminology tapes of a speaker pronouncing a list of medical terms may also be helpful to international/ESL students.
- International/ESL students must be able to differentiate important versus unimportant information in the test questions.
- Use tapes with content and test questions to help incorporate the information.
- Be aware of culturally bound words or words that have several different meanings. Ask for clarification from a faculty member.
- Tape lectures and listen to them several times.
- Tape questions and answers from NCLEX-PN® test banks. Include the rationale for the correct answer. Then listen to the tapes several times.
- After reading a test question, visualize the scenario before reading the options.

NCLEX® Contact Information

NCLEX® Candidate Services

United States
(Toll free) (866)-49-NCLEX or (866) 496-2539
  Monday through Friday; 7 a.m. to 7 p.m., US Central Time

Asian Pacific Region
Call NCLEX Candidate Services in Sydney, Australia: (Toll) +61.2.9478.5400
  Monday through Friday; 7 a.m. to 7 p.m., Australian Eastern Time

Europe, Middle East, Africa
Call NCLEX Candidate Services: (Toll) +44.161.855.7455
  Monday through Friday; 8 a.m. to 6 p.m., Central European Time

India
Call NCLEX Candidate Services: (Toll) 91.120.439.7837
  Monday through Friday; 9 a.m. to 6 p.m., IST

All Other Countries
(Toll) (952) 681-3815
  Monday through Friday; 7 a.m. to 7 p.m., U.S. Central Time

Nursing Process

- **Assessment:** Participate in collecting client data relevant to the client's health status.
- **Diagnosis:** Participate in the analysis of collected data by recognizing existing relationships among client data, client health status, and treatment regimen.
- **Planning:** Participate in developing the client's plan of care; assist in establishing appropriate client interventions and outcomes.
- **Implementation:** Deliver nursing care according to an established health care plan within the scope of nursing practice.
- **Evaluation:** Participate in determining the extent to which desired outcomes of nursing care have been met and in planning for subsequent care.

Leadership and Management

Leadership styles of nursing leadership include:

- **Autocratic:** A dictatorship; does not involve others in the decision-making process
- **Democratic:** Participative leadership; encourages others to participate in the decision-making process
- **Laissez-faire:** Permissive management; allows employees to make all decisions
- **Multicratic or participative:** A compromise between the autocratic and democratic leader; provides structure appropriate to the situation and encourages maximum group participation

Management Functions

Management functions performed by licensed practical nurses include:

- **Planning:** Helping to develop a plan of care
- **Organizing:** Providing an orderly environment that promotes cooperation and goal achievement

- **Directing:** Making assignments to unlicensed personnel
- **Coordinating:** Looking at a situation to ensure that it is being handled in the most effective way
- **Controlling:** Evaluating the accomplishment of the organization's goals
- **Delegating:** Empowering unlicensed persons to perform client care tasks when qualified

Delegation Process

To effectively delegate, the nurse must:

- Know the state practice act rules for delegation
- Match the skills and talents of the delegate to the task being delegated

---

National Council of State Boards of Nursing Five Rights of Delegation:

1. Right task
2. Right circumstances
3. Right person
4. Right communication
5. Right supervision

Legal Considerations

Standard of Care

Acceptable nursing standards of care include:

- **Duty to seek medical care for the client:** It is the legal duty of the nurse to ensure that every client receives safe and competent care.
- **Confidentiality:** The Health Insurance Portability and Accountability Act (HIPAA) of 1996 ensures that all client information, including medical records, is confidential.
- **Permission to treat:** Upon admission to a facility, clients must sign a legal document that gives health care providers permission to treat them.

- **Informed consent:** Informed consent is a process of communication between a physician and a client that results in the client's signed authorization to undergo a specific medical intervention. It is the responsibility of the physician to ensure that the client fully understands the risks and benefits of the intervention and alternatives to treatment.
- **Defamation of character:** The act of sharing information that is malicious and false. When the defamation is written, it is called libel. When the defamation is oral, it is called slander.
- **Advanced directives:** The Patient Self-Determination Act ensures that a person has an opportunity to make decisions regarding health care in advance of an illness or a need for treatment that would prohibit making such critical decisions.
- **Negligence:** Negligence occurs when a person fails to perform according to established standards of care. Malpractice is negligence by a professional person with a license.
- **Fraud:** Fraud is deliberate deception for the purpose of personal gain.
- **Assault:** Assault is the threat of unlawful touching of another or the willful attempt to harm someone.
- **Battery:** Battery can mean any of the following:
  - The unlawful touching of another without consent, justification, or excuse
  - False imprisonment
  - Preventing movement or making a person stay in a place without obtaining consent, either through physical or nonphysical means

Ethical Considerations

Nursing Code of Ethics

The National Association for Practical Nurse Education and Service (NAPNES) developed an LPN/LVN code of ethics.

Ethical Principles

The following ethical principles relate to nursing practice:

- **Autonomy:** The right of self-determination, independence, and freedom
- **Beneficence:** The principle of taking action to benefit another

- **Fidelity:** The obligation to be faithful to commitments made to self and others
- **Veracity:** The virtue of truthfulness
- **Nonmaleficence:** The principle of not harming the client, either intentionally or unintentionally
- **Justice:** The ethical principle that people of similar circumstances or conditions should be treated alike

Ethical Decision-Making

The steps involved in ethical decision-making include:

- Gathering information
- Clarifying the values of all the participants
- Identifying the ethical dilemma and the conflicts in values
- Examining possible actions and the consequences of each action
- Determining the standard of best interest
- Planning the best action with the strongest ethical support
- Implementing the action
- Evaluating the outcome

Communication

Types of Communication

Nursing communication includes the following types:

- **Nonverbal:** Gestures, body language, and facial expression
- **Verbal:** Words, phrases, or sentences
- **Failed:** Misinformation, misinterpretation, or improper documentation; a primary cause of medication errors
- **Feedback:** A response to an action or idea; can be positive or negative
- **Assertive:** Expressing one's feelings or asserting one's rights while respecting the feelings and rights of others
- **Aggressive:** Expressing one's feelings or asserting one's rights in a disrespectful, demeaning, or abusive manner
- **Passive:** Failing to communicate one's own feelings to "keep the peace"
- **Passive-Aggressive:** Inability to express anger in a healthy way; abusive

Communication Principles for the Clinical Setting

Nursing communication principles include the following:

- Think before you speak.
- Be quiet and gentle in your communication.
- Ask only appropriate questions.
- Do not talk about clients or their families in inappropriate places.
- Be respectful in your communication with others.
- Seek information in the least intrusive manner possible.

Therapeutic Communication

Technique	Description	Example
Encouraging descriptions of perceptions	Asking the client what he or she is seeing or hearing	"Tell me what the voices are saying to you."
Encouraging comparison	Asking the client to compare similarities or differences	"How is the medication working for you compared with the last time you used it?"
Exploring	Looking deeper into a subject, idea, or experience	"Tell me more about the last time you were depressed."
Focusing	Concentrating on a single idea or event	"Tell me more about how your divorce made you feel."
Formulating a plan of action	Assisting the client to come up with a plan to cope with stress	"When this happens in the future, how could you handle it more constructively?"
Giving broad openings	Allowing the client to steer the interaction	"What would you like to work on today?"
Giving recognition	Acknowledging or showing awareness	"I see that you brushed your hair today."

Continued

Therapeutic Communication—*cont'd*

Technique	Description	Example
Making observations	Verbalizing what is observed	"I notice you seemed upset after your wife visited."
Offering self	Extending one's presence	"I am available to talk whenever you would like."
Offering general leads	Giving the client encouragement to continue	"I see...."
Placing event in time or sequence	Clarification of events in time	"Was this before or after your first hospitalization?"
Presenting reality	Defining reality in simple terms	"The voices may seem real to you, but they are a symptom of your illness."
Restating	Repeating the main idea of what the client has verbalized	"It sounds as if you are feeling frustrated."
Reflecting	Statements, questions, or feelings are referred back to the client	"What do you think you should do?"
Seeking clarification	Searching for understanding of what was said	"Tell me if this is what you meant when you said..."
Verbalizing the implied	Putting into words what the client has implied or said indirectly	"You must be feeling very sad right now."
Using silence	Giving both the nurse and the client a chance to collect their thoughts and organize what they are going to say	

Communication Barriers

Mechanism	Description	Example
Agreeing/ disagreeing	Implies that the nurse has the right to pass judgment on whether the client's ideas or opinions are "right" or "wrong"	"That is right on target. I agree 100%."
Asking "Why" questions	Implies that the client knows the reason for his or her behavior and feelings	"Why were you feeling so angry?"
Changing the subject	Takes control of the conversation away from the client	Client: "I am feeling so hopeless." Nurse: "Did you go to group therapy today?"
Giving advice	Implies that the nurse knows what is best	"I think you should..."
Giving approval or disapproval	Passes judgment on the client's ideas or opinions	"That's right."
Giving false reassurance	Devalues the client's feelings	"Everything is going to be all right."
Engaging in self-focusing behavior	The nurse focuses on his or her own feelings at the expense of the client's	"That happened to me once...let me tell you about it."
Giving double-bind messages	The nonverbal message doesn't match the verbal message	"I am listening," as the nurse fidgets in her chair, doesn't make eye contact, and then coughs.

Teaching/Learning Principles

Client Factors That Influence Learning

Culture, Religion, Ethnicity, and Language
- Be culturally sensitive and nonjudgmental.
- Avoid assumptions, biases, and stereotypes. Seek help from the multicultural team.
- Use a professional translator.

Knowledge and Experience
- Identify what the client already knows. Build on this foundation.
- Explore concerns related to experiences. Correct misconceptions.

Literacy
- Assess the client's ability to read and comprehend material.
- Provide privacy.

Developmental Level

Children
- The younger the child, the shorter the attention span.
- Toddlers and preschoolers are concrete thinkers; school-age children are capable of logical thinking.
- Use a direct and simple approach; include the child's parents.

Adolescents
- Be open and honest about illness.
- Respect opinions and the need to be accepted by peers.
- Support his or her need for control.
- Learning must have immediate results.

Adults
- Learning is most effective when self-directed, is built on prior knowledge and experience, and has a perceived benefit.

Older Adults
- Functional changes, stress, fatigue, and chronic illness can decrease learning.
- Changes that may occur include slower cognition, slower reaction time, becoming overwhelmed with too much detail, and decreased ability to recall new information.

Readiness to Learn

- Client has to recognize the need to learn and be physically and emotionally able to participate.
- Depression, anxiety, anger, and denial can interfere with readiness, motivation, and concentration.
- Pain, acute/chronic illness, oxygen deprivation, fatigue, weakness, and sensory impairment can interfere with learning.
- Select teaching aids appropriate for client's sensory limitations.
- Postpone teaching until client is able to focus on learning; address factors that interfere with learning.

Motivation

- Assess client's personal desire to learn.
- Ensure material is meaningful.
- Identify/praise progress; allow for mistakes.
- Use interactive strategies; do not allow anxiety level to increase beyond mild anxiety.

Nutrition and Diet Therapy

Food Pyramid Guidelines

Food Groups	Serving Sizes	Recommended Behavioral Change
Bread, Cereal, Rice, and Pasta (6-11 servings/day)	• 1 slice of bread • 1 oz of ready-to-eat cereal • ½ cup of cooked cereal, rice, or pasta	• Use whole grain products; eat oatmeal or bran cereal daily. • Eat at least 1/2 cup of dried beans, peas, or lentils daily.
Vegetable (minimum of 5 servings/day)	• 1 cup of raw, leafy vegetables • ½ cup of other vegetables, cooked or chopped raw • ¾ cup of vegetable juice	• Choose one reliable source of vitamin A daily (green or orange vegetable, such as carrots, sweet potatoes, winter squash, spinach, or broccoli). • Include one serving of a green, leafy vegetable daily.

Continued

Food Pyramid Guidelines—cont'd

Food Groups	Serving Sizes	Recommended Behavioral Change
Fruit (minimum of 4 servings/day)	• 1 medium apple, banana, orange • ½ cup of chopped, cooked, or canned fruit • ¾ cup of fruit juice	• Choose one or two reliable sources of vitamin C daily (orange juice or fruit; grapefruit juice or fruit, cantaloupe, strawberries). • Eat one serving of a red or purple fruit or vegetable daily (tomatoes, blueberries, strawberries). • Eat whole fruit and avoid fruit with added sugars.
Milk, Yogurt, and Cheese (3 servings/day)	• 1 cup of milk or yogurt • 1–1½ ounces of natural cheese • 2 oz of processed cheese	• Use nonfat or very low-fat dairy products.
Meat, Poultry, Fish, Dry Beans, Eggs, and Nuts (Maximum of 6 oz/day)	• 2–3 oz of cooked lean meat, poultry, or fish • ½ cup of cooked dry beans or 1 egg counts as 1 oz of lean meat; 2 tbsp of peanut butter or ⅓ cup of nuts counts as 1 oz of meat.	• Select lean meat and cut off all visible fat before cooking. • Use soy and soy products as meat substitutes. • Weekly eat one serving of a fatty fish (e.g., salmon, tuna, herring, swordfish).
Other (eat sparingly)		• Eat one tsp of ground flax seed daily. • Include one clove of garlic and onion daily. • Use olive, peanut, and canola oil

Religious/Cultural Customs that Affect Food Intake

Religion/Culture	Restricted Food/Beverages and Cultural Practices
African American	• Food is cooked with a lot of saturated fats.
Buddhism	• All meat is prohibited.
Catholicism	• Meat is prohibited on Ash Wednesday and Fridays during Lent.
Chinese	• Rice and wheat are main staples.
Hinduism	• Beef, pork, and some fowl are prohibited.
Hispanic	• Foods are stewed or fried in oil. • Sugar is added to foods. • Corn is the main staple.
Islam	• Avoid all pork and pork products, carnivorous animals, birds of prey, and land animals without external ears. • Avoid meat not slaughtered according to ritual. • No blood or blood by-products. • No alcohol or intoxicants.
Native American	• Consume taro, sweet potatoes, breadfruit, fruit, greens, and seaweed. • Food consumed is high in fat and sugar.
Orthodox Judaism	• Avoid all pork and pork products; all fish without scales and fins. • Dairy products are not eaten at the same meal with meat and meat products. • Meat is slaughtered according to ritual, thoroughly draining the blood, which is forbidden. • Bakery products and food mixtures are prepared under acceptable kosher standards. • Leavened bread and cake are forbidden during Passover. • If kosher meal is unavailable, a cottage cheese and fruit plate is a good choice.
Seventh-Day Adventist	• Avoid all pork and pork products, shellfish, all flesh foods, dairy products and eggs, blood, meat broths, highly spiced foods, coffee, and tea.

Life Cycle Nutrition

Life Cycle	Nutritional Requirements	Nutritional Problems
Pregnancy	• 10 g protein per day to build fetal tissue • Folic acid is required • 3-4 mg of iron per day during third trimester • 3.5–4.5 servings of milk or milk products per day • 1 mg fluoride • 3 servings of meat or meat substitute per day provide enough zinc caloric increases during pregnancy: 200–300 calories per day the 2nd and 3rd trimesters	• Alcohol predisposes fetus to fetal alcohol syndrome. • Caffeine affects fetal heart rate and breathing patterns. • Raw or contaminated milk, soft cheeses, contaminated vegetables, and ready-to-eat meats can cause listeriosis infections. • Infants of women who smoke have increased risk of perinatal mortality. • Infants of women with cocaine addiction suffer from immature mental development.
Breast-feeding mothers	• Additional 2 milk exchanges; 1 meat exchange; 1 fruit or vegetable high in vitamin C; increase in fluid intake of 1 L/day	• Human lactation is associated with alterations in calcium metabolism that are independent of dietary intake and unresponsive to increase in calcium intake.
Infancy	• Breast milk is natural for human infants. • Breast milk contains more amylase than cow's milk.	• Honey should not be given until after the first birthday. • Feeding honey increases risk of allergies.

Continued

Life Cycle	Nutritional Requirements	Nutritional Problems
Infancy (cont'd)	• Infant needs 30%–55% of kilocalories from fat. • Cow's milk contains nine times the vitamin B_{12} of breast milk. • Breast milk contains more vitamin C, but less vitamin D, than cow's milk. • Breast milk contains less sodium, potassium, chloride, phosphorus, calcium, and iron than cow's milk. • Breast milk contains more zinc than cow's milk and formula.	• Breast milk is a cause of *Lactobacillus* organisms, which contribute to infant mortality. • Delay egg whites until age 1 year. • Iron-deficiency anemia is caused by drinking too much milk. • Foods that produce allergic reactions include milk, eggs and egg whites, nuts, peanut butter, oranges, orange juice, wheat protein, and chocolate.
Toddler	• Expected weight gain of 4–6 lbs. per year • Introduce unmodified cow's milk, egg white, wheat, citrus fruits, seafood, chocolate, and nut butters after first birthday. • Small serving size is recommended (1 tbsp = 1 serving). • Provide daily serving of vitamin C–rich fruit or vegetable and green leafy or yellow vegetable. • Increase fiber. • Offer three meals and three nutritious snacks.	• Limit sugar consumption. • Discourage consumption of heavily salted foods. • Limit milk to 24 oz/day.

Continued

Life Cycle Nutrition — cont'd

Life Cycle	Nutritional Requirements	Nutritional Problems
Preschool child	• Expected weight gain of 4–5 lbs. per year. • 3-year-old may need 1300–1500 Kcal/day. • Serving size for 4–6-year-olds is same as for adults. • Needs three meals and three nutritious snacks. • Wholesome snacks should be available.	• Concentrated sweets and soda pop should be strictly limited. • Emphasize brushing teeth after meals. • American Academy of Pediatrics recommends supplements only for children at nutritional risks.
School-age child	• Adult balanced diet is good for school-age child. • Breakfast is an important meal. • Provide variety, balance, and moderation. • Liberal intake of milk and milk products before age 10 years. • Moderation of sodium intake is indicated for girls younger than age 11 years.	• Lack of a balanced diet leads to overweight children. • Increase of diabetes is found with sedentary lifestyles and obesity.
Adolescent	• This age group may require 60–80 Kcal/kg of body weight/day. • Athletic teens need B vitamins.	• Two common nutritional problems in teens are anorexia/bulimia and poor choices of food.
Mature adult	• Aging affects all body systems, thus affecting nutrition.	• Fewer than 50% of women consume the recommended serving of any food group.

Dietary Management for Symptom Control

Anemia

- Recommend a vitamin C source with red meats and iron-fortified foods.
- Discourage intake of coffee, tea, and chocolate if client has gastrointestinal bleeding.
- Recommend multivitamin supplement, but avoid megadoses of vitamins.

Anorexia

- Suggest small, frequent feedings.
- Educate to recognize early signs of malnutrition, provide protein supplements, make food accessible, and encourage eating as desired by the client.
- Evaluate client acceptance of a liquid diet and recommend complete oral nutritional supplements.

Bowel Obstruction

- NPO is indicated for complete bowel obstruction.
- Provide intravenous feedings as indicated.

Cachexia

- Teach relaxation techniques and encourage their use before mealtimes.
- Concentrate on the sensual pleasures of eating, such as setting an attractive table and plate and removing environmental distractions.

Constipation

- Recommend an increased intake if needed.
- Encourage high-fiber foods (bran, whole grains, fruits, vegetables, nuts, and legumes) if adequate fluid intake can be maintained.
- Instruct to avoid high-fiber foods if dehydration or an obstruction is suspected or anticipated.
- Recommend limiting cheese and high-fat, sugary foods that may be constipating.
- Discontinue calcium and iron supplements if contributing to constipation.

Cough
- Encourage fluids and ice chips.
- Recommend hard candy.
- Try caffeinated tea and coffee to dilate pulmonary vessels.

Dehydration
- Encourage fluids, such as juices, ice cream, gelatin, custards, puddings, and soups.
- Encourage trying creative beverages, such as orange sherbet floats and milkshakes.
- If necessary, plain water and foods high in electrolytes can be delivered via a tube feeding.

Diarrhea
- Consider modification of diet to omit lactose, gluten, or fat if related to diarrhea.
- Recommend a decrease in dietary fiber content.
- Consider the use of a low-residue diet.
- Encourage high-potassium foods (bananas, tomato juice, orange juice, potatoes, etc.) if dehydrated.
- Recommend dry feedings (drink fluids 1 hour before or 30 to 60 minutes after meals).
- If client has pancreatic insufficiency, encourage a diet high in protein and carbohydrates.
- Consider the use of a complete oral nutritional supplement to provide adequate nutrient composition, while helping the client overcome mild-to-moderate malabsorption.
- For copious diarrhea and/or diarrhea combined with a decubitus on the coccyx, consider the use of a clear liquid diet.
- Recommend a complete nutritional supplement.

Dyspnea
- Encourage caffeinated coffee, tea, carbonated beverages, and chocolate to break up and expel pulmonary secretions and fluids.
- Encourage use of a soft diet. Liquids are usually better tolerated than solids. Cold foods are often better accepted than hot foods.
- Recommend small, frequent feedings.
- Encourage ice chips, frozen fruit juices, and popsicles.
- Consider the use of a complete high-fat, low-carbohydrate nutritional supplement.

Esophageal Reflux

- Recommend small feedings.
- Discourage foods that reduce esophageal sphincter pressure, such as high-fat foods, chocolate, peppermint, spearmint, and alcohol.
- Encourage client to sit up while eating and for 1 hour afterward.
- Recommend avoidance of food within 3 hours before bedtime.
- Teach relaxation techniques.

Fever

- Recommend a high-fluid intake.
- Consider a tube feeding for severe dehydration to maintain hydration.
- Recommend high-protein, high-caloric foods.

Fluid Accumulation

- Evaluate need for sodium restriction.
- Evaluate protein and potassium intake and encourage increased intake, if appropriate.

Hypoglycemia

- Assess the client's and/or caregiver's knowledge about diabetes and hypoglycemia.
- Assess if client is insulin dependent.
- Determine the last time the client experienced the signs of a hypoglycemic episode.
- Monitor client's blood glucose level.
- Encourage 30–50 g of carbohydrate every 3 hours to prevent starvation ketosis.
- Evaluate the need for specialized oral nutritional supplements for clients with liver disease.

Nausea and Vomiting

- Restrict fluids to 1 hour before or after meals.
- Recommend avoidance of sweet, fried, or fatty foods, if poorly tolerated.
- Encourage starchy foods, such as crackers, breads, potatoes, rice, and pasta, if tolerated.
- Encourage the client to eat slowly, chew food well, and rest after each meal.
- Recommend avoiding food preparation areas if food odors induce nausea.

- Recommend one or two bites of food per hour if extremely nauseated.
- Recommend the avoidance of food if nausea and vomiting become severe and food makes the client feel worse.

Stomatitis (Inflammation of the Mouth)

- Consider a multivitamin supplement with folic acid and vitamin B_{12}.
- Recommend avoidance of spicy, acidic, rough, hot, and salty foods.
- Recommend a consistency modification, such as pureed, soft, or liquid.
- Consider the use of a complete nutritional supplement.
- Recommend creamy foods, white sauces, and gravies.
- Consider between-meal supplements, such as milkshakes, eggnogs, and puddings.
- Recommend adding sugar to acidic or salty foods to alter the food's taste.
- Recommend meals be served when the client's pain is under control.
- Recommend good oral care before and after meals.

Weakness

- Recommend a multivitamin–mineral supplement with folic acid, vitamin B_{12}, and iron.
- Encourage high-potassium foods if client vomits easily.
- Recommend a modification in the food's consistency (mechanical soft or full liquid) to decrease the energy cost of eating.

Wounds and Pressure Sores

- Start nutrition intervention early (oral supplements and/or peripheral nutrition).
- Consider the client's food preferences.
- Correct elevated glucose levels to decrease risk of infection.
- Recommend avoidance of extremely hot or cold foods.
- Recommend creamy foods, white sauces, and gravies.
- Encourage the client to dip foods in gravy, margarine, butter, olive oil, coffee, and broth.
- Consider the need for a complete liquid nutritional supplement between meals.

I. Improve the Accuracy of Client Identification

- Use at least two client identifiers before administering medications, taking blood samples and other specimens, or providing any treatments or procedures.
- Identify the client by using the client's date of birth, full name, or medical record number from the client's armband.
- **NEVER use the client's room number as an identifier.**
- Prior to the start of any invasive procedure, perform a final verification to confirm the correct client, procedure, site, and availability of appropriate documents.
- Use active, not passive, communication techniques to verify the client's identity.

II. Improve the Effectiveness of Communication Among Caregivers

- Read back the entire order or critical test result when receiving information verbally or by telephone.
- Refer to a standardized list of abbreviations, acronyms, and symbols that are NOT to be used within the organization.
- Report critical test results and values in a timely manner.
- Use a standardized approach to "hand off" communications when transferring client care; take time to ask and answer questions.

III. Improve the Safety of Using Medications

- Label all medications, medication containers (e.g., syringes, medicine cups, basins) and other solutions on or off the sterile field.
- Annually review the organization's list of look-alike/sound-alike drugs; take action to prevent errors involving these drugs.
- Use caution when administering any medication, especially high alert medications.

IV. Reduce the Risk of Health-Care–Associated Infections

- Prevent nosocomial infections (those that are acquired in the health-care setting); take action to prevent infections resulting from multiple drug-resistant organisms.
- Use WHO and CDC hand hygiene guidelines.
- Use standard (universal) precautions and transmission-based precautions when needed.
- Report unanticipated deaths or permanent loss of function from nosocomial infections as "sentinel events."
- Use best practices to prevent central line–associated bloodstream infections and surgical site infections.

V. Accurately and Completely Reconcile Medications During Care

- Obtain a complete list of the client's current medication upon admission.
- Compare the client's current medications to those ordered within the organization.
- Communicate the complete list of client medications to the next health-care provider within or outside of the organization.

VI. Reduce the Risk of Client Harm From Falls

- Follow organizational guidelines to prevent falls.
- Keep bed rails up and keep client call bell within easy reach.

VII. Reduce the Risk of Influenza and Pneumococcal Disease

- Follow organizational recommendations for administration of flu vaccine and *pneumococcus* vaccine, especially for institutionalized older adults.
- Report new cases promptly and help to manage outbreaks.

VIII. Reduce the Risk of Surgical Fires

- Obtain education about risks for surgical fires if working in the surgical area.

IX. Encourage Client Involvement in Own Care as Safety Strategy

- Identify ways that the client and his or her family can express concerns about safety and encourage communication of concerns.

X. Prevent Health-Care–Associated Pressure Ulcers

- Collect data regarding each client's risk for developing pressure ulcers (decubitus ulcers) and take action to address any identified risk.
- Report suspected ulcers to RN and recheck affected area frequently.

XI. Identify Safety Risks Inherent to Client Population

- Identify and report clients who may be at risk for suicide.
- Identify and report risks associated with oxygen administration (i.e., risk of home fire).

XII. Improve Recognition and Response to Changes in Client's Condition

- Report any changes in client's condition to RN or other health-care team member, especially if the client's condition is worsening.

XIII. Use Universal Protocols

- Verify the client's identity before any procedure.
- Mark the procedure side/site when preparing the client; have client write his or her initials on the procedure side/site if possible.
- Perform a "time out" immediately before a procedure to verify client identity, procedure to be performed, and marked side/site of procedure.

Source: The Joint Commission. (2009). National Patient Safety Goals for Hospitals. Available at: http://www.supportingsaferhealthcare.com/2008/12/2009-joint-commission-national-patient-safety-goals-for-hospitals-.html.

Safety: Administering Oxygen

Caution: Highly Flammable
Always place a "No Smoking" sign on client's door
and over bed when using oxygen.

Nasal Cannula

- Used for low flow, low % of oxygen.
- Delivers 22%–44% oxygen.
- Flow rate of 1–6 L/min.
- Client can eat, drink, and talk.
- Use humidifier with extended use; check level of sterile, distilled water.
- Change cannula daily.

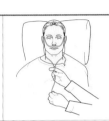

Simple Face Mask

- Used for higher percentages of oxygen.
- Delivers 35%–60% oxygen.
- Flow rate of 6–10 L/min.
- Side perforations allow CO_2 to escape.
- Permits humidification; check level of sterile, distilled water often.

Exhalation ports

Elastic strap

To oxygen source

Venturi Mask

- Used for precision titration of percentage of oxygen.
- Delivers 24%–40% oxygen.
- Flow rate of 4–8 L/min.
- Accurate delivery of O_2 by setting dial to % oxygen to be delivered.
- Change mask, tubing, and nebulizer daily.
- Drain tubing often to remove water condensation that has formed.

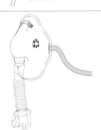

Reading Pulse Oximeters

Finding	Intervention
$SpO_2 > 95\%$	• Considered normal. • No intervention required. • Continue to monitor client.
SpO_2 91% to 94%	• Considered acceptable. • Assess probe placement and adjust as needed. • Continue to monitor client.
SpO_2 85% to 90%	• Raise head of bed and stimulate client to breathe deeply. • Encourage coughing and reposition client. • Reposition probe to a different location to rule out false reading. • Notify RN. • Assist RN in notifying physician and respiratory therapist if SpO_2 fails to improve after a few minutes.
$SpO_2 < 85\%$	• Notify RN immediately. • Reposition client to facilitate breathing. • Assist RN as needed. • Be prepared to manually ventilate if condition worsens or fails to improve.

■ The reliability of pulse oximeters is sometimes questionable.
■ Many conditions may produce false readings:
  ▪ Anemia: False high
  ▪ Hypovolemia: False high
  ▪ Client movement: Erratic readings
  ▪ Cool extremities: False low
  ▪ Nail polish: False low
  ▪ Poor peripheral circulation: False low
  ▪ Certain vasoconstrictors: False low

Notify team leader or RN immediately if interventions fail to increase SpO_2 level after a few minutes or if client is experiencing distress.

Safety: Client Positioning

Purpose
To prevent undue stress on the musculoskeletal system, enhance client comfort, and prevent injury to the client

Guidelines
- Position clients who are weak, frail, in pain, paralyzed, or unconscious in good body alignment to promote client comfort and safety.
- **Keep bedrails up and call bell within easy reach at all times.**
- Reposition clients every 2 hours.
- Use support devices, such as pillows, mattresses, bed boards, chair beds, and footboards to position clients.
- Administer pain medication, if indicated, prior to moving the client.
- Plan around encumbrances, such as IVs, indwelling catheters, casts, etc.

Common Client Positions	
Position	**Description**
Fowler's position	Semi-sitting with head of bed elevated 45 to 90 degrees
Semi-Fowler's position	Semi-sitting with head of bed elevated 15 to 45 degrees
High-Fowler's position	Sitting with head of bed elevated to 90 degrees
Orthopneic position	Sitting on side of bed with tray table across lap; facilitates respirations
Supine position	Back-lying with head and shoulders on small pillow; also called dorsal recumbent position
Prone position	Lying on abdomen with head turned to one side; used only for short periods
Lateral position	Side-lying with top hip and knee flexed and supported; good for resting and sleeping; relieves pressure from sacrum and heels
Sims' position	Semi-prone position; halfway between lateral and prone with pillow under head, upper arm, and upper leg; good for pregnant women and clients who are unconscious to facilitate mouth drainage

Safety: Chest Drainage Systems

Purpose

To drain fluid or air from the pleural space

Types of Systems

Glass Bottle System:

- Water Seal Bottle:
  - Each time the client exhales, air trapped in the pleural space travels through the chest tube into the water seal bottle.
  - The water acts as a seal, preventing air from re-entering the pleural space during inspiration.
  - Water in the tube rises during inspiration and falls during expiration, which is called **tidaling**.
- Glass Suction Bottle:
  - A suction source used to speed lung inflation.
  - Usually set at negative 20 cm of water.
  - Suction should be turned on far enough to cause gentle bubbling.
- Glass Drainage Bottle:
  - Catches fluid drained from pleural space.
  - Drainage level in bottle is marked and timed, not emptied.
  - Drainage should be recorded as output.

Molded Plastic System:

- Works the same as bottle system.
- Some one-piece systems have valves, eliminating the need for water.

Chest Tube Care:

- Observe respiratory rate, effort, symmetry, shortness of breath, and pain; observe for tidaling.
- Confirm that dressing is intact; observe for drainage.
- **DO NOT change the dressing;** reinforce dressing and notify RN or physician if necessary.
- Report bloody drainage to RN; mark amount of drainage in collection chamber every 8 hours or as ordered.
- Notify RN or physician if client reports suddenly increasing dyspnea or if the drainage chamber is full and needs to be changed.

- Keep drainage system upright and below level of client's chest; ensure that there are no dependent loops of tubing.
- **DO NOT strip or milk chest tube to dislodge clots**.

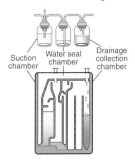

Suction chamber · Water seal chamber · Drainage collection chamber

Safety: Nasogastric/Orogastric Tubes

Purpose
To remove gas and fluids from the stomach (decompression); to diagnose GI motility; to relieve and treat obstructions or bleeding; to provide nutrition; to remove toxic substances; to promote healing after upper GI surgery

Types of Tubes
- **Orogastric tube:** GI tube that is inserted through the mouth and into the stomach
- **Nasogastric tube:** GI tube that is inserted through the nares into the stomach

Tube Care
- Ensure that tube is secured in place with tape; provide daily skin care to taped area to prevent skin breakdown.
- Slipknot a rubber band around tube and fasten to client's gown.
- Provide frequent oral care to keep mucous membranes moist.
- Prevent excessive intake of ice chips if suction is used to prevent electrolyte imbalance.

■ Flush every 2 to 4 hours to maintain patency; use only normal saline to prevent electrolyte imbalance.
■ Record accurate I&O.

Safety: Nasogastric Tube Feedings

Purpose
To provide oral nutrition and/or medications when the GI system is functioning but the PO route is unavailable

Types of Tube Feedings
■ **Initial Tube Feeding:** Advance feedings as tolerated by 10 to 25 mL/hr every 8 to 12 hours until goal rate is reached
■ **Intermittent Tube Feedings:** Infusions of 200 to 400 mL of enteral formulas infused over 30-minute periods several times daily
■ **Continuous Feedings:** Feedings that are administered over 24 hours with the use of an infusion pump

Tube Feeding Guidelines
Confirm Placement Prior to Using
■ Inject a 20-mL bolus of air into the feeding tube while auscultating the abdomen; loud gurgling indicates proper placement.
■ **DO NOT** confirm tube placement by using water!
■ Gently aspirate gastric contents using a 20-mL syringe; dip litmus paper into gastric aspirate; a pH of 1 to 3 suggests proper placement.
■ X-ray is the most reliable method of verifying tube placement.

Maintenance
■ Flush with 30 mL of water every 4 to 6 hours, before and after tube feedings, checking residuals, and medication administration.

Medication
■ Dilute liquid medications with 20 to 30 mL of water.
■ Obtain all medications in a liquid form; if not available, then check with pharmacy to see if medication can be crushed.
■ Administer each medication separately and flush with 5 to 10 mL of water between medications.
■ **DO NOT** mix medications with feeding formula!

Residuals

- Check before bolus feedings, administration of medication, or every 4 hours for continuous feeding.
- Hold feeding if residual is >100 mL and recheck in 1 hour.
- If residuals are still high after 1 hour, notify RN or physician.
  - **To check residuals:**
    - Use a 60-mL syringe to aspirate any residual formula that may remain in the stomach.
    - Note the volume of the residual; if more than the predetermined amount, then withhold next feeding.
    - A greater than expected residual volume means that the stomach is not emptying properly, which may indicate gastroparesis and/or intolerance to the advancement of formula feedings.

Safety: Restraints

Definition
A restraint is any physical or pharmacological method of restricting a client's movements, activities, or access to his or her body.

Uses
Restraints should be used only as a last alternative after all other methods of control have been attempted; can only be used to prevent clients from harming themselves or others or to prevent the client from interfering with necessary medical treatments; may never be used for discipline or staff convenience.

Guidelines
Requires a written physician order that must be renewed every 24 hours. Order must specify the clinical necessity, type of restraint, frequency of assessment, and duration of time the restraint is to be used. **Always refer to facility policies and procedures when using restraints.**

Applying Restraints
- Obtain informed consent from client or family.
- Verify written physician order.
- Check skin, circulation, sensation, and motion of area before applying restraint.
- Client should be restrained in an anatomically correct position with bony prominences padded to prevent pressure sores.

- Always follow manufacturer's instructions when applying restraints.
- Apply the restraint loosely enough for two fingers to fit under the restraint.
- Restraints should be secured to bed frame or chair using quick-release knots.
- **Never attach a restraint to the bedrail**.
- Call bell must be easily accessible to client.
- Check restraint sites every 15 minutes.
- Remove restraints every 2 hours if possible.
- Document findings and interventions after each check.
- Report findings to team leader or RN.

Safety: Suctioning

Preparation
- Prepare the client; explain procedure; offer reassurance.
- Gather and set up supplies and equipment.
- Wash hands; use standard precautions.
- Position self at client's bedside so that nondominant hand is toward the client's head.
- Preoxygenate client with 100% O_2 for several deep breaths.

Nasal or Oral Suctioning
Purpose
To remove secretions and maintain airway clearance; to stimulate deep cough reflex.

Guidelines
- If oxygen is in use, remove before suctioning and replace immediately after.
- Depth required for proper nasal suctioning in the adult is 20 cm.
- To verify correct length, measure from nose to ear and ear to mid sternum.
- If resistance is met during suctioning, release suction pressure.
- If resistance is met passing the catheter, do not force.
- Document color, amount, and consistency of secretions.
- Document client response to suctioning.

Endotracheal or Tracheostomy Tube Suctioning:
Purpose
To remove secretions and maintain a patent airway; to stimulate cough reflex.

Guidelines
- Document client response to suctioning, including respiratory status, before and after suctioning.
- Don sterile gloves and insert sterile suction catheter just far enough to stimulate cough reflex.
- Apply intermittent suction while withdrawing catheter and rotating 360 degrees for no longer than 10 to 15 seconds to prevent hypoxia.
- Ventilate client with 100% oxygen for several deep breaths.
- Repeat until client's airway is clear, rinsing catheter in sterile saline between attempts.
- Suction oropharynx after suctioning airway.
- Document color, amount, and consistency of secretions.
- If secretions are thick and difficult to remove, 5 to 10 mL of sterile saline may be instilled before hyperoxygenation with an Ambu® bag.
- If necessary, have another nurse present to help with procedure.

Infection Control

Four categories of microorganisms cause infection in humans:

- **Bacteria:** The most infection-causing microorganisms.
- **Viruses:** Common virus families include the rhinovirus (common cold), hepatitis, herpes, and human immunodeficiency virus (HIV).
- **Fungi:** Includes molds and yeasts, such as *Candida albicans*.
- **Parasites:** Live on other organisms; examples are protozoa (which cause malaria), helminths (worms), and arthropods (mites, fleas, and ticks).

INFECTION CONTROL: 2007 CDC STANDARD AND TRANSMISSION-BASED PRECAUTIONS

Tier I: Standard (Universal) Precautions

Indications: Recommended for care of <u>all</u> clients regardless of their diagnosis or infection status

Purpose: To provide a barrier protection for all health care providers; to prevent the spread of infectious disease

Application: To be used when coming in contact with blood, body fluids (except sweat), secretions, excretions, nonintact skin, and mucous membranes

Types of Standard Precautions

Hand washing: The single most important means of preventing the spread of disease. Perform before and after every client contact and after contact with blood, body fluids, or contaminated equipment.

Gloves: Nonlatex gloves should be worn whenever contact with body fluids is possible. Note: Lotions may degrade gloves.

Mask and eye protection: Worn whenever splashing by body fluids is possible or in the presence of airborne infections.

Gown: Worn whenever exposed skin or clothing may become soiled during client contact or when contact precautions are implemented.

Disposal of Sharps: Needles and other sharp instruments should be disposed of in a labeled, puncture-resistant biohazard container. **Never re-cap needles.**

Containment: Soiled linens should be placed in a leak-proof bag. Grossly contaminated refuse should be placed in a red biohazard bag and placed in an appropriate receptacle.

Decontamination: Contaminated equipment should be properly disinfected per facility guidelines. Single-use equipment should be properly disposed of after use.

Tier II: Transmission-Based Precautions (Used in Addition to Standard Precautions)

Airborne Precautions: Used for clients with known or suspected illnesses transmitted by droplet nuclei smaller than 5 microns.

Specific precautions include: Private room, negative airflow (at least six changes per hour), mask. Client may need to wear mask if coughing.

Used for: Measles, chicken pox, disseminated varicella zoster, tuberculosis (Tb).

Droplet Precautions: Used for clients with known or suspected illnesses transmitted by droplet nuclei greater than 5 microns.

Specific Precautions: Private room, mask. Client may need to wear mask if coughing.

Used for: *Haemophilus influenzae* type B and *Neisseria meningitidis* (meningitis, pneumonia, sepsis), diphtheria, pertussis, streptococcal pharyngitis, scarlet fever in children, adenoviruses, mumps, rubella.

Contact Precautions: Used for clients with known or suspected illnesses transmitted by contact with client or by contact with items in the client's environment.

Specific Precautions: Private room, gloves, and gown; client may need to wear mask if coughing excessively.

Used for: Infection with drug-resistant bacteria, GI, respiratory, skin, and wound infections, *Clostridium difficile, Escherichia coli, Shigella,* hepatitis, rotavirus, respiratory syncytial virus (RSV), diphtheria, herpes simplex, impetigo, scabies, pediculosis, and others.

Infection Control: WHO Hand Washing Guidelines

Purpose
To prevent the spread of infection

World Health Organization (WHO) Guidelines
- Wash hands with soap and water under a stream of water for at least 20 seconds when visibly dirty, when contaminated with blood or body fluids, or after using restroom.
- Use an alcohol-based hand rub for routine hand asepsis if hands are not visibly soiled.
- Perform hand hygiene:
  - Before and after client contact.
  - After removing gloves.
  - Before handling an invasive device.
  - After contact with mucous membranes, nonintact skin, or wound dressings.
  - After contact with items in the vicinity of the client.
  - Before handling medication or preparing food.

- Antimicrobial soaps are recommended in high-risk areas.
- DO NOT wear artificial fingernails or extensions when having direct contact with clients.
- Keep natural nails short (less than 0.5 cm long).
- Educate clients and families on the importance of hand washing.

Most Common Infections

Location	Common Sources
Urinary Tract	
Escherichia coli	Improper catheterization technique, feces, colostomies
Pseudomonas aeruginosa	Improper hand washing, urinary diversion
Bloodstream	
Hepatitis B virus	Sexual contact, needle stick, IV drug use
Human immunodeficiency virus (HIV)	Sexual contact, needle stick, IV drug use
Staphylococcus aureus	Improper IV site care, open wound
Staphylococcus epidermis	Open wound, nonintact skin or mucous membrane
Lung (Pneumonia)	
Staphylococcus aureus	Improper hand washing
Parainfluenza virus	Sneezing, coughing, breathing
Mycobacterium tuberculosis	Sneezing, coughing, breathing
Surgical Sites	
Staphylococcus aureus (including methicillin-resistant [MRSA] strains)	Improper hand washing, drainage from incision
Enterococcus species (including vancomycin-resistant [VRE] strains)	Improper dressing change, drainage from incision
Pseudomonas aeruginosa	Improper dressing change
Gastrointestinal Tract	
Hepatitis A virus	Ingestion of contaminated food
Salmonella species	Ingestion of contaminated food
Clostridium difficile	Mouth, anus, ostomies

Signs and Symptoms of Infection

Increased pulse, respirations, and WBCs
Nodes are enlarged
Function is impaired
Erythema, edema, and exudate
Complains of discomfort/pain
Temperature—local and systemic

Infection Control: Asepsis

Purpose
To decrease the possibility of transferring microorganisms from one place to another; asepsis means "no infection"

Types
- **Medical asepsis:** Confining the growth of microorganisms to a specific area; limiting the number, growth, and transmission of microorganisms
- **Surgical asepsis:** Sterile technique; keeping an area or object free of all microorganisms

Principles of Asepsis
- Ensure that objects are cleaned, disinfected, or sterilized before use.
- Change dressings and bandages when they are soiled or wet.
- Dispose of damp, soiled linens appropriately.
- Ensure that all containers, such as bedside water pitchers and suction/drainage bottles, are covered or capped.
- Empty suction/drainage bottles at the end of each shift or according to agency policy.
- Wash hands between client contacts, after touching bodily substances, before performing invasive procedures, and before and after wound care.
- Use standard or transmission-based precautions as indicated.
- Use sterile technique when exposing open wounds or changing dressings.
- Use sterile technique for invasive procedures (e.g., injections, catheterizations, IV insertion).

- Place used disposable needles and syringes in puncture-resistant containers.
- Maintain the integrity of the client's skin and mucous membranes.
- Provide all clients with their own personal care items.
- Check to see if healing is taking place by determining whether wound secretions and size are decreasing and whether granulation is taking place.
- Check with RN regarding giving pain medication before wound care.
- Be careful when sitting the client up in the bed to prevent a possible shearing force.
- Avoid massage of sites of stage 1 pressure ulcers.

Infection Control: Ostomy Care

Purpose
To collect fecal material leaving the client's body through the abdomen

Types of Ostomies
- **Colostomy:** May be permanent or temporary; used when part of the large intestine is removed; commonly placed in the sigmoid colon; stoma is made from large intestine and is larger in appearance than an ileostomy; contents range from firm to fully formed, depending on the amount of intact intestine
- **Ileostomy:** May be permanent or temporary; used when entire large intestine is removed; stoma is made from small intestine; contents range from pastelike to watery
- **Urostomy:** Used when urinary bladder is either bypassed or removed

Ostomy Care Guidelines
To change an ostomy bag follow these guidelines:

- Wash hands and use standard precautions.
- Place client in supine position and remove old pouch by gently pulling away from skin.
- Discard gloves, wash hands, and don a new pair of gloves.
- Gently wash area around stoma with warm, soapy water; dry skin thoroughly.
- Inspect appearance of stoma and the condition of the skin; note the amount, color, consistency, and odor of contents.

- Cover the exposed stoma with a gauze pad to absorb any drainage during ostomy care.
- Apply skin prep in circular motion and allow to air dry for 30 seconds.
- Apply skin barrier in circular motion; measure stoma using stoma guide and cut ring to size.
- Remove paper backing; using gentle pressure, center the ring over the stoma and press into place; smooth out any wrinkles to prevent seepage of effluent.
- Center faceplate of bag over stoma and press down until completely closed.
- Document and discard soiled items per facility policy using standard precautions.

Infection Control: Urinary Catheters

Purpose
To drain the bladder and/or to collect urine specimens

Types of Catheters
- **Straight catheter:** Also called a "red rubber catheter" or "straight cath." Straight catheters are used to drain the bladder or to collect urine specimens. They only have a single lumen and do not have a balloon to hold them in the bladder.
- **Indwelling catheter:** Also called a Foley or retention catheter. Indwelling catheters have two lumens: one for urine drainage and another for inflation of the balloon near the tip, which holds the catheter in the bladder.

Catheter Care Guidelines
- Use standard precautions.
- Keep bag below level of client's bladder at all times.
- Do not tug or pull on catheter.
- Do not apply powder around insertion site.
- Perform complete perineal hygiene twice daily with soap and water to prevent bladder infection (more often if area becomes contaminated with stool or appears reddened, irritated, or swollen).
- Observe and document condition of urinary meatus.
- Note character of urine and report foul odor, cloudy appearance, or sediment.

- Empty catheter drainage bag every 8 hours, when full, or when transporting client.
- Document urine output every shift or per physician order.
- Immediately report to RN:
  - Blood, cloudiness, or foul odor
  - Urine output of less than 30 mL/hour
  - Irritation, redness, swelling, tenderness, or drainage around insertion site
  - Fever or abdominal or flank pain.

Infection Control: Vaccines/Immunizing Agents

Purpose
Immune globulins provide passive immunization to infectious diseases by providing antibodies. Immunization with vaccines and toxoids containing bacterial or viral antigenic material should result in endogenous production of antibodies.

Guidelines
- Measles, mumps, and rubella vaccine; trivalent oral polio; and diphtheria toxoid, tetanus toxoid, and pertussis vaccine may be given concurrently.
- Administer each immunization by appropriate route.
- Inform client/parent of potential and reportable side effects of immunization. Health-care professional should be notified if client develops fever higher than 39.4°C (103°F); difficulty breathing; hives; itching; swelling of the eyes, face, or inside of nose; sudden severe tiredness or weakness; or convulsions.
- Review next scheduled immunization with client/parent. Emphasize the importance of keeping a record of immunizations and dates given.

Administration
- IM
- PO

Infection Control—Wound Care

Purpose
To prevent infection, to assist in healing smaller wounds, and to prevent tetanus

Considerations
- Expect a variety of infection types from wounds exposed to standing water, sea life, and ocean water.
- Wounds in contact with soil and sand can become infected.
- Puncture wounds may carry bits of clothing and dirt into wounds and result in infection.
- Crush injuries are more likely to become infected than wounds from cuts.
- Evaluate whether client has received a tetanus immunization within the last 5 years.

Wound Care Guidelines
- Wash hands thoroughly with soap and clean water.
- Use standard precautions.
- Avoid touching the wound with your fingers while treating it (if possible, use disposable, latex gloves).
- Remove obstructive jewelry and clothing from the injured part.
- Apply direct pressure to any bleeding wound to control bleeding.
- Clean the wound after bleeding has stopped.
- Examine wounds for dirt and foreign objects.
- Gently flood the wound with bottled water or saline solution.
- Gently clean around the wound with soap and clean water.
- Pat dry and apply an adhesive bandage or dry clean cloth.
- Leave unclean wounds, bites, and punctures open.
- Wounds that are not cleaned correctly can trap bacteria and result in infection.
- Document location of wound and record drainage or moisture on outside of dressing that was removed.
- Check for any fresh blood on dressing.
- Assess client for pain; administer pain medication as ordered.

Bomb Threat/Event

In the event of a bomb threat:

- Leave the area immediately; Call **911**. Tell the operator what you saw or know (suspicious persons, packages, or vehicles).
- Follow directions from people in authority.
- Follow existing evacuation guidelines.

If involved in a bombing event:

- Leave the area immediately.
- Avoid crowds. Crowds of people may be targeted for a second attack.
- Avoid unattended cars and trucks. Unattended cars and trucks may contain explosives.
- Stay away from damaged buildings to avoid falling glass and bricks. Move at least 10 blocks or 200 yards away from damaged buildings.
- Follow directions from people in authority (police, fire, EMS, military personnel, or school or workplace supervisors).
- Call **911** once you are in a safe area but only if police, fire, or EMS has not arrived.
- Help others who are hurt or need assistance to leave the area if you are able. If you see someone who is seriously injured, seek help.

When the explosion is over:

- Follow your family, job, or school emergency disaster plan for leaving and staying away from the scene of the event.
- Avoid crowds. Crowds of people may be targeted for a second attack.
- Avoid unattended cars and trucks. Unattended cars and trucks may contain explosives.
- Stay away from damaged buildings.
- Follow directions from people in authority.
- Call **911** once you are in a safe area.
- Help others who are hurt or need assistance to leave the area.
- Listen to your radio or television for news and instructions.

Seek medical attention for the following problems:

- Excessive bleeding
- Trouble breathing
- Persistent coughing
- Trouble walking or using arm or leg
- Stomach, back, or chest pains
- Headache
- Blurred vision or burning eyes
- Dry mouth
- Vomiting or diarrhea
- Rash or burning skin
- Hearing problems
- Injuries that increase in pain, redness, or swelling
- Injuries that do not improve after 24 to 48 hours

Biological Agents

Anthrax
- **Etiology:** Caused by exposure to *Bacillus anthracis*.
- **Transmission:** Cutaneous and inhalation.
- **Onset:** Within 7 days; most cases occur within 48 hours; inhalation may take up to 6 weeks.
- **Signs and Symptoms:** Flulike symptoms (fever, muscle aches, cough, chest pain) progressing to respiratory distress and shock. Cutaneous anthrax results in a boil-like lesion that forms as an ulcer with a black center.
- **Treatment:** Obtain specimens for culture before initiating antimicrobial therapy. Treat with ciprofloxacin or doxycycline. Do not use extended-spectrum cephalosporins or trimethoprim/sulfamethoxazole because anthrax may be resistant to these drugs.
- **Precautions:** Standard contact precautions. Avoid direct contact with wound or wound drainage. A vaccine is available only to people in high-risk areas such as military personnel.
- **Prognosis:** Cutaneous requires prompt attention; inhalation is usually fatal if not treated immediately.

Botulism

- **Etiology:** Caused by *Clostridium botulinum*; results in muscle paralysis.
- **Transmission:** By eating contaminated food.
- **Onset:** Symptoms usually begin within 12 and 36 hours after eating contaminated food.
- **Signs and Symptoms:** Double or blurred vision, drooping eyelids, slurred speech, dry mouth, difficulty swallowing, muscle weakness that begins in the shoulders and arms and descends through the body. Paralysis of diaphragm leads to respiratory arrest.
- **Treatment:** Antitoxin is available and reduces severity if administered early; no vaccine is available.
- **Precautions:** Standard precautions; not spread from person to person.
- **Prognosis:** Most clients recover after weeks of supportive care.

Plague

- **Etiology:** Bacterial; caused by *Yersinia pestis*.
- **Transmission:** Person-to-person contact and by direct contact with body fluids and contaminated objects; may be intentionally dispersed in an aerosol form.
- **Onset:** 1 to 3 days for inhaled aerosol exposure; 2 to 8 days for fleaborne transmission.
- **Signs and symptoms:** Fever, cough, chest pain, headache, hemoptysis, leukocytosis.
- **Treatment:** First line: doxycycline; second line: ciprofloxacin. Clients are contagious until 72 hours of antibiotic treatment has been completed; no vaccine available.
- **Precautions:** Standard precautions.
- **Prognosis:** Fatal if not treated.

Smallpox

- **Etiology:** Viral; variola virus.
- **Transmission:** Person-to-person contact and by direct contact with body fluids and contaminated objects; client is contagious until lesions have scabbed over and fallen off (approximately 3 weeks).
- **Onset:** 7 to 17 days; average onset is 12 days.
- **Signs and symptoms:** Skin lesions appear, quickly progressing from macules to papules to vesicles; most prominent on head and extremities, whereas chicken pox is most prominent on the trunk; fever, myalgia, rash.

- **Treatment:** Supportive care; a vaccine is available.
- **Precautions:** Standard precautions.
- **Prognosis:** 30% fatality rate.

Chemical Agents

Decontamination

Should be performed within the first minute or two of exposure:

- To prevent the chemical from being further absorbed by the body or spreading on the body.
- To prevent the chemical from spreading to other people who must handle or who might come in contact with the person who is contaminated with the chemical.

If exposed to a dangerous chemical:

- Remove clothing; if clothing has to be pulled over head, then cut it off instead of pulling it over head; try to avoid touching any contaminated areas if helping others and remove the clothing as quickly as possible.
- Wash any chemicals from the skin with large amounts of soap and water. If eyes are burning or vision is blurred, rinse the eyes with plain water for 10 to 15 minutes. Remove contact lenses and put them with the contaminated clothing. Do not replace contacts. Wash eyeglasses with soap and water.
- Dispose of clothes. Use rubber gloves or tongs to put clothes into a biohazard bag. Seal the bag and then place sealed bag inside another bag (double bag).
- Dress in clean clothes; avoid coming in contact with other people who have been exposed and not yet washed and changed clothes.

Mustard Gas

- **Transmission:** Skin contact, eye contact, inhalation; not communicable.
- **Onset:** 2 to 24 hours after exposure.
- **Signs and symptoms:** Itching followed by blistering, irritation of eyes, runny nose, epistaxis, sneezing, hoarseness, coughing, and shortness of breath.

■ **Treatment:** Remove residue from body by blotting and then washing with soap and water; treat effects as clinically indicated; no antidote is available.
■ **Precautions:** Standard precautions.
■ **Prognosis:** Usually not fatal.

Sarin Gas

■ **Transmission:** Skin contact, eye contact, inhalation, ingestion; not communicable after decontamination.
■ **Onset:** Within seconds of exposure.
■ **Signs and symptoms:** Runny nose, sweating, blurred vision, headache, difficulty breathing, drooling, nausea and vomiting, increased urination, increased defecation, muscle spasms and twitching, confusion, convulsions, paralysis, coma.
■ **Treatment:** Administer antidote; atropine 2 to 6 mg IM. Remove from source; remove and double bag clothing; wash skin with soap and water; irrigate eyes for 10 to 15 minutes; do not induce vomiting.
■ **Precautions:** Standard precautions, contact precautions, airborne precautions.
■ **Prognosis:** Can be fatal within 15 minutes of exposure.

VX Nerve Agent

■ **Transmission:** Skin contact, eye contact, inhalation, ingestion possible but unlikely.
■ **Onset:** Within seconds to hours of exposure.
■ **Signs and symptoms:** Runny nose, sweating, blurred vision, headache, difficulty breathing, drooling, nausea and vomiting, increased urination, increased defecation, muscle spasms and twitching, confusion, convulsions, paralysis, coma.
■ **Treatment:** Administer antidote; atropine 2 to 6 mg IM. Remove from source; remove and double bag clothing; wash skin with soap and water; irrigate eyes for 10 to 15 minutes; do not induce vomiting.
■ **Precautions:** Standard precautions, contact precautions, airborne precautions; clothing can release VX for 30 minutes after exposure.
■ **Prognosis:** Mild/moderate exposure: usually recover within 1 to 2 weeks; severe exposure is usually fatal.

Medication Administration

Causes of Medication Errors

- Failed communication, such as poorly written orders, verbal orders, ambiguous and incomplete orders.
- Sound-alike/look-alike drugs.
- Misuse of zeroes in decimal numbers.
- Use of apothecary measures (grains, drams) or package units (amps, vials, tablets) instead of metric measures (grams, milligrams, milliequivalents).
- Misinterpreted abbreviations.
- Poor distribution practices, such as dispensing multidose floor stock vials instead of unit doses.
- Dose miscalculations.
- Drug packaging and drug delivery system failures.
- Incorrect drug administration.
- Lack of client education.

Five Medication Rights
1. Right client
2. Right medication
3. Right dose
4. Right time
5. Right route

Safety Check

- Check label when obtaining medication from storage.
- Perform side-by-side comparison of the medication with the written order and the medication administration record (MAR).
- Recheck one last time after preparation, just before administration.
- If giving heparin or insulin, double-check dosage with another nurse before and after drawing up medication.

Approximate Onset of Medication

■ Intravenous (IV): 3–5 min.
■ Intramuscular (IM): 3–20 min.
■ Subcutaneous (SC): 3–20 min.
■ Oral (PO): 30–45 min.

Assessment

■ Assessment needs vary depending on route and type of medication.
■ Always assess client after giving drugs that affect heart rate, B/P, level of consciousness, blood sugar, and pain.
■ Certain drugs require assessment of heart rate or blood pressure prior to giving medication.

Precautions

■ If blood appears in the syringe, withdraw the needle, discard the syringe, and prepare a new injection.
■ Do **not** aspirate or massage site when giving SC injections; bleeding inside tissue may occur.
■ Always confirm compatibility.
■ Always check for allergies and assess for reactions to drugs.
■ Always check to see what type of over-the-counter medications and herbal supplements the client is taking.
■ **Do not crush time-release or enteric-coated capsules or pills**.
■ Take vital signs (VS) before and 5 minutes after applying nitroglycerin (NTG) paste.
■ Always change the needle after withdrawing medication from a glass ampule.
■ Use a straw when you administer oral (PO) iron to prevent staining the teeth.
■ When giving SC injections, if less than 1 inch can be pinched between fingers, then pinch skin and insert needle at a 45-degree angle; if more than 1 inch can be pinched, spread the skin and insert at a 90-degree angle.
■ Be certain that medications mixed in the same syringe are compatible. A cloudy appearance noted in the syringe after mixing may indicate incompatibility.

Common Medication Abbreviations					
AC	Before meals	kg	Kilogram	Q 2 hr	Every 2 hours
AU	Each ear	mcg	Micrograms	QID	4 times per day
BID	Twice a day	mEq	Milliequivalent	Rect	Rectally
cap	Capsule	mg	Milligram(s)	Subcu	Subcutaneous
ER	Extended release	mL	Milliliter(s)	tab(s)	Tablet(s)
gm	Gram	NKA	No known allergies	Tbs	Tablespoon
gtt	Drop	OD	Right eye	TID	3 times daily
ID	Intradermal	OS	Left eye	tsp	Teaspoon
IM	Intramuscular	OU	Both eyes	VO	Verbal order
IV	Intravenous	PO	By mouth	X	Times (e.g., x2)

Source: Deglin, J. & Vallerand, A. (2009). *Davis's Drug Guide for Nurses* (11th ed.). Philadelphia: F.A. Davis Company.

Common Medication Calculations

I. Basic Formula:

$$\frac{\text{Desired dose}}{\text{On-hand amount}} \times \text{Quantity} = \text{Answer}$$

Example: A physician orders hydromorphone 1.5 mg IV every 4 hours for pain. The dose on hand is hydromorphone 2 mg/5 mL. How much medication should a nurse give to the client?

$$\frac{1.5 \text{ mg}}{2.0 \text{ mg}} \times 5 \text{ mL} = \frac{7.5}{2.0} = \textbf{3.75 mL}$$

II. Volume per Hour (IV Pumps):

$$\frac{\text{Total mL ordered}}{\text{Total time ordered in hours}} = \text{mL/hour (rounded to a whole number)}$$

Example: A physician orders 1,000 mL of fluid to be infused intravenously over a period of 2 hours. At what rate should a nurse set the infusion pump?

$$\frac{1,000 \text{ mL}}{2 \text{ hours}} = \textbf{500 mL/hr}$$

III. Drops per Minute (Manual IV Sets):

$$\frac{\text{Total volume} \times \text{Drip set factor (gtts)}}{\text{Total time (minutes)}} = \text{Rate of flow}$$

Example: A physician assistant orders 1,000 mL normal saline to be infused intravenously over a period of 24 hours. At how many drops per minute should the nurse infuse the solution?

$$\frac{1,000 \text{ mL} \times 20 \text{ gtts}}{24 \text{ hrs (60)}} = \frac{20,000 \text{ mL}}{1,440 \text{ min}} = 13.88 = \textbf{14 gtts/min}$$

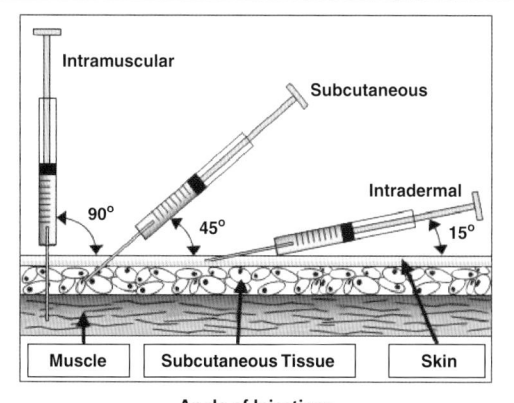

Angle of Injections

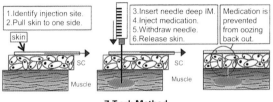

Z-Track Method

Insulin Injections

Types of Insulin				
Course	**Agent**	**Onset**	**Peak**	**Duration**
Rapid-acting insulins	Insulin lispro (Humalog®)	5 min	60–90 min	4–6 hr
	Insulin aspart (NovoLog®)	10–20 min	1–3 hr	3–5 hr
Short-acting insulins **Caution: Regular insulin is the *only* insulin that can be given IV by RN.**	Regular insulin (Humulin R®)	**SC route:** 30–60 min **IV route:** 10–30 min	**SC route:** 2–4 hr **IV route:** 15–30 min	**SC route:** 5–7 hr **IV route:** 30–60 min
	Concentrated insulin (Insulin U-500) **Caution: Do not give IV.**	30–60 min	2–3 hr	5–7 hr
Intermediate-acting insulins	NPH (Humulin N®, Novolin R®)	1–2 hr	8–12 hr	18–24 hr
Long-acting insulins	Insulin glargine (Lantus®) **Caution: Cannot be mixed with other insulins**	Onset: 1 hour. Provides a constant concentration over a 24-hr period with no pronounced peak.		
	Insulin detemir (Levemir®)	2–4 hr	None	24 hr

Types of Insulin—cont'd

Course	Agent	Onset	Peak	Duration
Premixed insulins	NPH/Regular (Humulin 50/50®, Humulin 70/30®), (Novolin 70/30®)	30–60 min	2–9 hr	24 hr
	Aspart Protamine/ Aspart (NovoLog Mix 70/30®)	10–20 min	2 ½ hr	24 hr
	Lispro protamine/ Lispro (Humalog Mix 75/25®)	5 min	2 hr	22 hr

- Remember to triple-check all medication orders for insulin and have another nurse present when you mix the insulin; insulin is a high-alert medication.
- Insulin should be administered SC with the needle at a 45-degree angle.
- Do not aspirate or massage site when administering SC insulin.
- Each insulin injection should be spaced at least 1 inch from the previous injection.
- Because each area absorbs insulin at a different rate, use one area for a week and then move to the next area.
- The torso (abdomen and buttocks) provide the most uniform absorption.
- When mixing insulins, always draw up the clear insulin first.

The Evens-and-Odds Rule

To remember the onset, peak, and duration of insulins:

- Think *evens* for intermediate-acting insulins: 2, 12, and 24 hours.
- Think *odds* for short-acting insulins: 1, 3, and 5 hours.

(Times are approximate.)

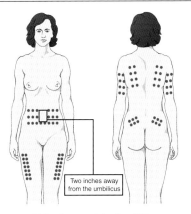

Two inches away
from the umbilicus

Subcutaneous Injection Sites

Mixing Insulin

Use only an insulin syringe. Start by withdrawing enough air into an insulin syringe that is equal to the combined amount of the total dose of insulin to be given. Without actually dipping the needle into the NPH solution itself, pressurize the NPH vial with the amount of air equal to the amount of NPH to be mixed with the regular insulin, and then remove the syringe.

U-100

Regular

Inject the remaining air into the regular insulin vial, and then withdraw the ordered amount of regular insulin into the syringe.

Regular

After withdrawing the ordered amount of regular insulin, remove the syringe, and expel any air bubbles.

NPH

Reinsert the syringe into the already pressurized NPH vial and withdraw the ordered amount of NPH.

NPH

IV Administration

Key Points for Administration of IV Medications

- Provide an environment that maximizes safe and efficient administration of medications.
- Follow the five rights of medication administration.
- Verify the prescription or medication order before administering the drug.
- Select the appropriate sizes of syringes and needles.
- Determine the correct dilution, amount, and length of administration time as appropriate.
- Monitor for the following:
  - Drug infusion at regular intervals.
  - Irritation, infiltration, and inflammation at the infusion site.
  - Therapeutic range of drug levels.
  - Therapeutic response.
  - Renal function for adequate excretion of drug through the kidneys.
  - Allergies, drug interactions, and drug incompatibilities.
  - Intake and output.
  - Need for pain relief medications.
- Maintain IV access.
- Administer drugs at selected times.
- Note the expiration date on the medication container.
- Administer medication using the appropriate technique.
- Dispose of unused or expired drugs according to agency policy.
- Maintain strict aseptic technique.
- Sign for opioids and other restricted drugs according to agency protocol.
- Document medication administration and client responsiveness.

Starting an IV

- **Prepare the client:** Explain procedure, answer any questions, and reassure.
- **Gather equipment:** IV bag with primed tubing, sharps container, catheter, tape, tourniquet, and antiseptic swabs.
- **Organize supplies:** Tear tape, have primed tubing and sharps container within easy reach, and open 2 × 2 dressing.
- **Apply tourniquet:** Proximal to intended insertion site, either mid-forearm or above the elbow.
- **Locate vein:** Palpate with fingertips. To further enhance dilation, gently tap, apply heat or warm soak, and have client make a few fists or dangle arm below heart.
- **Cleanse site:** Using moderate friction, cleanse in a circular motion, moving outward from intended site.
- **Use standard precautions:** Put on gloves while waiting for cleansed area to dry. Avoid touching site once it has been prepared.
- **Apply traction:** In the direction opposite the catheter.
- **Position needle:** Bevel side up, 15–30 degrees. Hold the needle with the thumb and pointer finger in a way that allows for visualization of the flash chamber.
- **Insert needle:** Observe for "flash back" (or blood return) in the flash chamber.
- **Insert IV:** Lower catheter almost parallel to the skin, and insert the needle 1–2 mm more to ensure that the catheter has also entered the vein.
- **Advance the catheter:** By threading the catheter into vein while maintaining skin traction.
- **Release the tourniquet:** Apply digital pressure just above the end of the catheter tip while gently stabilizing the hub of the catheter.
- **Remove needle:** Discard into approved sharps container.
- **Initiate infusion:** Connect IV tubing, open clamp, and observe for free flow of IV fluid.
- **Secure catheter:** Tape catheter securely and apply sterile dressing per hospital policy and procedure.
- **Document:** Note gauge of catheter, time of insertion, and client response in medical record.

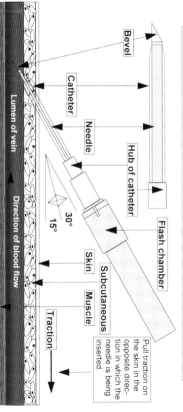

Notice how the catheter is slightly shorter than the needle. This is why the needle needs to be advanced 1–2 mm farther after the initial flash back and before advancing the catheter and removing the needle.

Bevel

Catheter

Needle

Hub of catheter

Flash chamber

30°

15°

Skin

Subcutaneous

Muscle

Traction

Lumen of vein

Direction of blood flow

Pull traction on the skin in the opposite direction in which the needle is being inserted.

Starting an IV

Management of Local IV Complications

Infiltration

SIGNS/SYMPTOMS: Swelling, tenderness, coolness of skin around site; decreased or no infusion rate; blanching of skin.

Treatment:
- Discontinue IV and restart in new site.
- Notify RN or team leader of complication.
- Apply warm compresses to the affected area.
- Elevate extremity if edematous.

Phlebitis

SIGNS/SYMPTOMS: Classic sign is red line along vein; redness, heat, swelling, tenderness.

Treatment:
- Discontinue IV and restart in new site.
- Notify RN or team leader of complication.
- Apply warm compresses to the affected area.
- Elevate extremity if edematous.

Hematoma

SIGNS/SYMPTOMS: Discoloration of skin; swelling; tenderness; inability to advance cannula all the way into vein; resistance to positive pressure.

Treatment:
- Discontinue IV and restart in new site.
- Notify RN or team leader of complication.
- Apply direct, light pressure with sterile 2 × 2 gauze for 2–3 minutes.
- Elevate extremity to maximize venous return.
- Apply ice to prevent further enlargement of hematoma.

Local Infection

SIGNS/SYMPTOMS: Swelling; tenderness; redness; possible exudate of purulent material; elevated temperature.

Treatment:

- Remove cannula and restart IV in new site.
- Notify RN or team leader of complication.
- Culture cannula and insertion site.
- Prepare at least two blood cultures before antibiotic therapy is initiated.
- Apply sterile dressing over site.
- Administer systemic antibiotic therapy as ordered.
- Continue to monitor site.

Management of Systemic IV Complications

Septicemia

SIGNS/SYMPTOMS: Fluctuating fever; tremors; profuse cold sweat; nausea and vomiting; diarrhea (sudden and explosive); abdominal pain; tachycardia; increased respirations; altered mental status; hypotension.

Treatment:

- Consult the physician.
- Restart a new IV in the opposite extremity.
- Obtain cultures from the administration set, container, catheter tip site, and the client's blood.
- Initiate antimicrobial therapy as ordered.
- Monitor the client closely.
- Determine whether the client's condition requires transfer to the ICU.

Fluid Overload and Pulmonary Edema

SIGNS/SYMPTOMS: Restlessness, headache; increase in pulse rate; weight gain over a short period of time; cough; presence of edema; hypertension; wide variance between intake and output; rise in central venous pressure (CVP); shortness of breath and crackles in lungs; distended neck veins.

Treatment:

- Consult the physician.
- Decrease the IV flow rate.

■ Place the client in high Fowler's position.
■ Keep the client warm to promote peripheral circulation.
■ Monitor vital signs.
■ Administer oxygen as ordered.
■ Consider changing the administration set to a microdrip set.

Air Embolism

SIGNS/SYMPTOMS: Palpitations; lightheadedness and weakness; dyspnea, cyanosis, tachypnea, expiratory wheezes, cough, and pulmonary edema; "mill wheel" murmur; weak, thread pulse; tachycardia; substernal chest pain; hypotension; and jugular venous distention; confusion, coma; anxiousness; seizures.

Treatment:
■ Notify the physician immediately.
■ Call for help.
■ Place the client in the Trendelenburg position on left side with the head down. This causes the air to rise in the right atrium, preventing it from entering the pulmonary artery.
■ Administer oxygen.
■ Monitor vital signs.
■ Call for emergency equipment
■ If untreated, these symptoms lead to death.

Medication Error—Intervention

■ **Discontinue the incorrect medication immediately!**
■ Notify RN or team leader promptly.
■ Observe for adverse drug reactions per facility protocol.
■ Notify physician of medication error and any adverse reactions to the medication.
■ Complete incident/variance report per facility protocol.
■ **Never** put a copy of an incident/variance report in a client's medical record.
■ **DO NOT** document that an incident/variance report was filed.

Recognizing an Adverse Drug Reaction (ADR):
- Type A reactions are predictable reactions based on the primary or secondary pharmacologic effect of the drug (i.e., dose-related reactions and drug–drug interactions).
- Type B reactions are unpredictable, are not related to dose, and are not the result of the drug's primary or secondary pharmacologic effect (i.e., hypersensitivity reactions):
  - Rash
  - Change in respiratory rate, heart rate, blood pressure or mental state
  - Seizure
  - Anaphylaxis
  - Diarrhea
  - Fever

Treatment of ADR:
- Determine that the drug ordered was the drug given as intended.
- Determine the drug was given in the correct dosage by the correct route.
- Establish the chronology of events: time drug was taken and onset of symptoms.
- Stop the drug and monitor client status for improvement.
- Restart the drug, if physician orders, and monitor closely for adverse reactions.

Documentation:
- Complete all appropriate documentation per facility protocol.
- Document on MAR and progress notes if indicated.
- Avoid using phrases such as "given in error." Document the medication, dose, time, and route on MAR.
- Document that the physician was notified.
- If an ADR occurs, document intervention and outcome.

Drug Classifications

Antianxiety Agents

PURPOSE: Management of various forms of anxiety, including generalized anxiety disorder.

Type	Action	Example
Benzodiazepines	Act at many levels of the CNS to produce anxiolytic effect; effects may be mediated by GABA, an inhibitory neurotransmitter.	Alprazolam (Xanax®) Diazepam (Valium®) Flurazepam (Dalmane®) Lorazepam (Ativan®) Midazolam (Versed®) Triazolam (Halcion®)
Serotonin reuptake inhibitors (SSRIs)	Inhibit neuronal reuptake of serotonin in the CNS thus potentiating the activity of serotonin.	Paroxetine (Paxil®) Fluoxetine (Prozac®) Sertraline (Zoloft®) Escitalopram (Lexapro®)
Miscellaneous	Alter the action of dopamine or norepinephrine in the CNS.	Buspirone (BuSpar®) Hydroxyzine (Atarax®) Venlafaxine (Effexor®)

Data Collection:
Baseline: CBC and differential; vital signs.

Implementation:
- SSRIs may take 1–4 weeks of therapy to obtain therapeutic effect.
- Monitor appetite and nutritional intake.
- Restrict amount of drug available to clients; psychological and/or physical dependence may occur.
- Weigh weekly; report continued weight loss.
- Monitor mental status.
- Report increases in anxiety, nervousness, or insomnia.
- Assess for suicidal tendencies, especially during early therapy.

ADMINISTRATION: PO or IV.

EVALUATION/DESIRED OUTCOME: Increased sense of well-being; renewed interest in surroundings; decrease in frequency and severity of panic attacks or episodes of anxiety.

Beta Blockers

PURPOSE: Management of hypertension, angina pectoris, tachyarrhythmia, hypertrophic subaortic stenosis, migraine headache (prophylaxis), MI (prevention), glaucoma (ophthalmic use), CHF (carvedilol and sustained-release metoprolol only), and hyperthyroidism (management of symptoms only).

Type	Action	Example
Beta blockers (nonselective)	Decrease myocardial oxygen consumption via a decrease in heart rate.	Carvedilol (Coreg®) Nadolol (Corgard®) Propranolol (Inderal®)
Beta blockers (selective)	Block stimulation of beta1 (myocardial) adrenergic receptors.	Acebutolol (Sectral®) Atenolol (Tenormin®) Metoprolol (Lopressor®)
Ophthalmic beta blockers	Decrease production of aqueous humor. Management of chronic open-angle glaucoma and other forms of ocular hypertension.	Carteolol (Ocupress®) Levobetaxolol (Betaxon®) Timolol (Timoptic®)

Data Collection:
Baseline: vital signs; intake and output ratios; daily weights; assess for signs of CHF (dyspnea, rales/crackles, weight gain, peripheral edema, jugular vein distention); laboratory tests: BUN, serum lipoprotein, potassium, triglyceride, uric acids, ANA titers, glucose, serum alkaline phosphatase, LDH, AST, ALT levels; EKG.

Implementation:
■ Instruct clients to continue taking medications, even if feeling well.
■ Encourage compliance with additional interventions for hypertension.

- instruct clients and families on proper technique of monitoring blood pressure.
- Caution clients to make position changes slowly to minimize orthostatic hypotension.
- Advise clients that exercising or hot weather may enhance hypotensive effects.
- Advise clients to consult health-care professional before taking any OTC medications or herbal/alternative therapies, especially cold remedies.
- Caution client that these medications may cause increased sensitivity to cold.
- Instruct diabetics to monitor blood glucose closely.
- Advise clients to report to health-care professionals their medication regimen prior to treatment or surgery.
- Advise clients to carry identification describing disease process and medication regimen at all times.
- Emphasize the importance of follow-up exams to monitor progress.

ADMINISTRATION: Beta blockers are given orally or via IM injection, IV, or eye drops.

EVALUATION/DESIRED OUTCOME: Decrease in blood pressure; decrease in frequency and severity of angina attacks; control of arrhythmias; prevention of myocardial infarction; prevention of migraine headaches; decrease in tremors; lowering of intraocular pressure.

Bone Resorption Inhibitors

PURPOSE: Used to treat and prevent osteoporosis in postmenopausal women. Other uses include treatment of osteoporosis from other causes, including corticosteroid therapy, treatment of Paget's disease of the bone, and management of hypercalcemia.

Type	Action	Example
Biphosphates	Inhibit resorption of bone by inhibiting hydroxyapatite crystal dissolution and osteo-clast activity.	Alendronate (Fosamax®) Etidronate (Didronel®) Ibandronate (Boniva®) Pamidronate (Aredia®) Risedronate (Actonel®)
Selective estrogen receptor modulators	Bind with estrogen receptors, producing estrogen-like effects on bone including decreased bone resorp-tion and decreased bone turnover.	Raloxifene (Evista®)

Data Collection:
Baseline: serum calcium, alkaline phosphatase, vital signs, electrolytes, hemoglobin, creatinine, CBC, platelet count, intake and output ratios, renal function, phosphate, and magnesium.

Implementation:
■ Assess clients for low bone density and periodically during therapy.
■ Assess clients for symptoms of Paget's disease (bone pain, headache, decreased visual and auditory acuity, and increased skull size).
■ Instruct clients to take medication exactly as directed.
■ Encourage clients to participate in regular exercise and to modify behaviors that increase the risk of osteoporosis.

ADMINISTRATION: May be given PO or IV.

EVALUATION/DESIRED OUTCOME: Prevention of or decrease in the progression of osteoporosis in postmenopausal client. Decrease in the progression of Paget's disease.

Bronchodilators

PURPOSE: Used in the treatment of reversible airway obstruction resulting from asthma or COPD.

Type	Action	Examples
Adrenergics	Produce bronchodilation by stimulating the production of cyclic adenosine monophosphate.	Albuterol (Proventil®) Epinephrine (EpiPen®) Formoterol (Foradil®) Levalbuterol (Xopenex®) Metaproterenol (Alupent®) Pirbuterol (Maxair®) Salmeterol (Serevent®) Terbutaline (Brethaire®)
Anticholinergics	Produce bronchodilation by blocking the action of acetylcholine in the respiratory tract.	Ipratropium (Atrovent®)
Leukotriene antagonists	Components of slow-reacting substance of anaphylaxis A (SRS-A), which may be a cause of bronchospasm.	Montelukast (Singulair®) Zafirlukast (Accolate®) Zileuton (Zyflo®)
Xanthines	Inhibit the breakdown of cyclic adenosine monophosphate.	Aminophylline (Phyllocontin®) Theophylline (Theobid®)

Data Collection:
Baseline: vital signs, monitor lung sounds, character of secretions before and after therapy, EKG, potassium levels, glucose levels, serum lactic acid concentrations, AST and ALT concentrations, ABGs, acid-base, fluid and electrolytes.

Implementation:
- Emphasize taking only the prescribed dose at the prescribed time intervals.
- Encourage clients to drink adequate liquids (2,000 mL/day minimum) to decrease the viscosity of the airway secretions.

- Instruct clients to avoid OTC cough, cold, or breathing preparations without consulting a health-care professional.
- Encourage clients to minimize intake of xanthine-containing foods or beverages (colas, coffee, and chocolate).
- Advise clients to avoid smoking and other respiratory irritants.
- Instruct clients on proper use of metered-dose inhaler.
- Instruct clients to contact a health-care professional promptly if the usual dose of medication fails to produce the desired results, symptoms worsen after treatment, or toxic effects occur.
- Clients using other inhalation medications and bronchodilators should be advised to use bronchodilator first and allow 5 min to elapse before administering the other medication, unless otherwise directed by health-care professional.

ADMINISTRATION: PO, inhalation, IV.

EVALUATION/DESIRED OUTCOME: Decreased bronchospasm and increased ease of breathing.

Calcium Channel Blockers

PURPOSE: Used in the treatment of hypertension, in the treatment and prophylaxis of angina pectoris or coronary artery spasm, in the treatment of arrhythmias, and to prevent neurologic damage from certain types of cerebral vasospasm.

Type	Action	Example
Calcium channel blockers	Block calcium entry into cells of vascular smooth muscle and myocardium. Dilate coronary arteries in both normal and ischemic myocardium and inhibit coronary artery spasm. Decrease AV conduction.	Amlodipine (Norvasc®) Diltiazem (Cardizem®) Nicardipine (Cardene®) Nifedipine (Procardia®) Nimodipine (Nimotop®) Nisoldipine (Sular®) Verapamil (Calan®)

Baseline: vital signs; intake and output; daily weights; ECG monitoring; total serum calcium levels; serum potassium levels; hepatic enzymes; nifedipine may cause positive ANA and direct Coombs' test results; platelet count.

Implementation:

- Teach clients not to open, crush, or chew sustained-release capsules.
- Instruct clients to take medication even if not feeling well.
- Caution clients to make position changes slowly to minimize orthostatic hypotension.
- Advise clients that exercising or hot weather may enhance hypotensive effects.
- Instruct clients on the importance of maintaining good dental hygiene.
- Advise clients to consult a health-care professional before taking any OTC medications or herbal/alternative therapies, especially cold remedies.
- Advise clients to carry identification describing disease process and medication regimen at all times.
- Instruct clients with angina taking concurrent nitrate therapy to continue taking both medications as directed and using SL nitroglycerin as needed for angina attacks.
- Encourage clients with hypertension to comply with additional interventions, such as weight reduction, low-sodium diet, regular exercise, smoking cessation, moderation of alcohol consumption, and stress management.
- Instruct clients and family members to check blood pressure weekly and report significant changes to a health-care professional.

ADMINISTRATION: PO, IV.

EVALUATION/DESIRED OUTCOME: Decrease in BP; decrease in frequency and severity of angina attacks; decrease in need for nitrate therapy; increase in activity tolerance and sense of well-being; suppression and prevention of supraventricular tachyarrhythmia; improvement in neurological deficits resulting from vasospasm following subarachnoid hemorrhage.

Central Nervous System Stimulants

PURPOSE: Used in the treatment of narcolepsy and as adjunctive treatment in the management of ADHD.

Type	Action	Example
Central nervous system stimulants	Produce CNS stimulation by increasing levels of neurotransmitters. Produce CNS stimulation. In children with ADHD, these agents decrease restlessness and increase attention span.	Amphetamine mixtures (Adderall®) Dexmethylphenidate (Focalin®) Dextroamphetamine (Dexedrine®, Dexostat) Methylphenidate (Ritalin®) Pemoline (Cylert®)

Data Collection:
Baseline: vital signs; weights biweekly; heights in children; plasma corticosteroid concentrations; CBC, differential, and platelet counts.

Implementation:
■ May produce false sense of euphoria and well-being. Provide clients with frequent rest periods and observe client for rebound depression after the effects of the medication have worn off.
■ These medications have a high dependence and abuse potential. Advise clients that abrupt cessation with high doses may cause extreme fatigue and mental depression.
■ Advise clients to avoid intake of large amounts of caffeine.
■ Medication may impair judgment. Caution clients to avoid driving or other activities requiring judgment until response to medication is known.
■ Inform clients that periodic holidays from the drug may be used to assess progress and decrease depression.

ADMINISTRATION: PO.

EVALUATION/DESIRED OUTCOME: Decreased frequency of narcoleptic episodes; improved attention span and social interactions.

Corticosteroids

PURPOSE: Used in replacement doses systematically to treat adrenocortical insufficiency. Larger doses are usually used for their anti-inflammatory, immunosuppressive, or antineoplastic effects.

Type	Action	Example
Inhalation	Used in the chronic management of reversible airway disease (asthma); potent, locally acting anti-inflammatory and immune modifier	Beclomethasone (QVAR®) Budesonide (Pulmicort®) Flunisolide (AeroBid®) Fluticasone (Flovent®) Triamcinolone (Azmacort®)
Nasal	Used in the management of chronic allergic and inflammatory conditions; potent, anti-inflammatory and immune modifier	Beclomethasone (Beconase®) Budesonide (Rhinocort®) Fluticasone (Flonase®) Mometasone (Nasonex®) Triamcinolone (Nasacort®)
Ophthalmic	Used in the management of inflammatory eye conditions including allergic conjunctivitis, nonspecific superficial keratitis, infectious conjunctivitis, management of corneal injury; suppression of graft rejection following keratoplasty, prevention of postoperative inflammation	Dexamethasone (Decadron®) Fluorometholone (Flarex®) loteprednol (Alrex®) Prednisone (AK-Pred®) Rimexolone (Vexol®)

Continued

Type	Action	Example
Systemic (short-acting)	Management of adreno-cortical insufficiency; chronic use in other situations is limited because of mineralocor-ticoid activity	Cortisone (Cortone Acetate®) Hydrocortisone (Solu-Cortef®)
Systemic (intermediate-acting)	Used systemically and locally in a wide variety of chronic diseases including inflammatory, allergic, hematologic, neoplastic, autoimmune disorders	Methylprednisolone (Solu-Medrol®) Prednisolone (Prednisol®) Prednisone (Deltasone®) Triamcinolone (Aristocort®)
Systemic (long-acting)	May be used as an alternate-day dosing in the management of chronic illness. May be used in the management of cerebral edema	Betamethasone (Celestone®) Budesonide (Decadron®) Dexamethasone (Decadron®)
Topical/local	Used as an anti-inflammatory, antipruritic, and vasoconstrictor. Application results in inhibition of macrophage/leukocyte migration as a result of decreased vascular dilation and per-meability. If systemically absorbed for prolonged periods, may produce adrenal suppression.	Alclometasone (Aclovate®) Amcinonide (Cyclosort®) Betamethasone (Diprosone®) Clocortolone (Cloderm®) Desoximetasone (Topicort®) Fluocinonide (Fluocin®) Hydrocortisone (Anusol HC®) Triamcinolone (Aristocort®)

Data Collection:

Baseline: assess for signs of adrenal insufficiency (hypotension, weight loss, weakness, nausea, vomiting, anorexia, lethargy, confusion, restlessness); height and weight of children; vital signs, especially respiration and lung sounds; adrenal function tests; serum urine glucose concentrations; check for glaucoma; intake and output ratios; daily weights; changes of levels of consciousness; serum electrolytes; serum glucose; hematologic values; guaiac-test stools; serum cholesterol levels; lipid levels.

Implementation:

- Teach signs of adrenal insufficiency.
- Instruct clients to eat a diet high in protein, calcium, and potassium and low in sodium and carbohydrates.
- Inform clients that these drugs cause immunosuppression and may mask symptoms of infection.
- Advise clients to avoid anyone who has a contagious illness and to report possible infections.
- Advise clients to consult health-care professional before receiving any vaccinations.
- Discuss possible effects on body image. Explore coping mechanisms.

ADMINISTRATION: Oral, injectable, topical, and inhalation; if dose is ordered daily or every other day, administer in the morning to coincide with the body's normal secretion of cortisol; when taking the drug orally, administer with meals to minimize gastric irritation.

EVALUATION/DESIRED OUTCOME: Suppression of the inflammatory and immune responses in autoimmune disorders, allergic reactions, and organ transplants; replacement therapy in adrenal insufficiency; resolution of skin inflammation, pruritis, or other dermatologic conditions.

Diuretics

PURPOSE: Enhances the selective excretion of various electrolytes and water by affecting renal mechanisms for tubular secretion and reabsorption.

Type	Action	Example
Loop diuretics	Used alone or in combination in the treatment of hypertension or edema resulting from CHF or other causes	Bumetanide (Bumex®) Furosemide (Lasix®) Torsemide (Demadex®)
Osmotic diuretics	Used in the management of cerebral edema	Mannitol (Osmitrol®)
Potassium-sparing diuretics	Have weak diuretic and antihypertensive properties and are used mainly to conserve potassium in clients receiving thiazide or loop diuretics	Amiloride (Midamor®) Spironolactone (Aldactone®) Triamterene (Dyrenium®)
Thiazide diuretics	Used alone or in combination in the treatment of hypertension or edema from CHF or other causes	Chlorothiazide (Diuril®) Chlorthalidone (thiazide-like) (Hygroton®) Hydrochlorothiazide (HydroDIURIL®)
Thiazide-like diuretics	Used alone or in combination in the treatment of hypertension or edema from CHF or other causes	Indapamide (Lozol®) Metolazone (Zaroxolyn®)

Data Collection:
Baseline: assess fluid status; daily weights; intake and output ratios; amount and location of edema; lung sounds; skin turgor; mucous membranes; signs of electrolyte imbalance (anorexia, muscle weakness, numbness, tingling, paresthesias, confusion, and excessive thirst); vital signs; neurological status and intracranial pressure readings; persistent

or increased eye pain or decreased visual acuity; lab tests (electrolytes, especially potassium, blood glucose, BUN, serum uric acid levels, serum cholesterol levels, low-density lipoprotein, and triglyceride concentrations.)

Implementation:

- Many diuretics are given in conjunction with antihypertensive medications.
- Caution clients to make position changes slowly to minimize orthostatic hypotension.
- Instruct clients to consult health-care professionals regarding potassium guidelines.
- Instruct clients to monitor weight weekly and report significant changes.
- Caution clients to use sunscreen and protective clothing to prevent photosensitivity reactions.
- Advise clients to consult health-care professionals before taking OTC medication concurrently with diuretics.
- Instruct clients to notify a health-care professional of medication regimen before treatment or surgery.
- Advise clients to contact a health-care professional immediately if muscle weakness, cramps, nausea, dizziness, or numbness or tingling of extremities occurs.
- Reinforce to clients the need to continue additional therapies for hypertension.
- Instruct clients with hypertension on the correct way of monitoring weekly blood pressures.

ADMINISTRATION: PO, IM, IV; administer oral diuretics in the morning to prevent disruption of the sleep cycle.

EVALUATION/DESIRED OUTCOME: Decreased blood pressure; increased urine output; decreased edema; reduced intracranial pressure; prevention of hypokalemia in clients taking diuretics; treatment of hyperaldosteronism.

Hormones

PURPOSE: Used in the treatment of deficiency states including diabetes, diabetes insipidus, hypothyroidism, menopause, and hormonally sensitive tumors.

Type	Action	Example
Hormones	Natural substances that have a specific effect on target tissue. Differ in their effect depending on individual agent and target tissue.	Calcitonin (salmon) (Calcimar®) Danazol (Danocrine®) Estrogens, conjugated (Premarin®) Fludrocortisone (Florinef®) Glucagon (GlucaGen®) Goserelin (Zoladex®) Insulins Levothyroxine (Synthroid®) Medroxyprogesterone (Depo-Provera®) Octreotide (Sandostatin®) Oxytocin (Pitocin®) Progesterone (Progestin®) Somatropin (Protropin®) Teriparatide (Forteo) Testerone (Andro®) Thyroid (Armour thyroid) Vasopressin (Pitressin®)
Contraceptive hormones	Synthetic substances used as contraceptive hormones and for symptoms of menopause.	Estradiol vaginal ring (Femring®) Ethinyl estradiol/drospirenone (Yasmin®) Ethinyl estradiol/etonogestrel (NuvaRing®) Ethinyl estradiol/norethindrone (Ortho-Novum 10/11®) Levonorgestrel (Norplant®) Medroxyprogesterone (Depo-Provera®)

Data Collection:

Baseline: vital signs; assess for signs and symptoms of hypoglycemia and hyperglycemia; serum inorganic phosphate, magnesium, and potassium levels; blood glucose and ketones; A1c may need to be monitored; assess client for bone pain; monitor intake and output ratios, assess for bladder distention; assess for endometrial pain; assess for symptoms of preco-cious puberty (menses, breast development, testicular growth); monitor testosterone, prostatic acid phosphate, and prostate-specific antigen (PSA); BUN, serum calcium, uric acid, hypoproteinemia, LDH, AST, hyper-lipemia, WBC, PT, or PTT, thyroid function tests; monitor children's height, weight, and psychomotor development; total cholesterol.

Implementation:

- Assess clients for signs of hormonal excess or deficiency.
- Monitor blood pressure and hepatic function tests periodically.
- Explain dosage schedule (and withdrawal bleeding with female sex hormones).
- Emphasize the importance of follow-up exams to monitor effective-ness of therapy and to ensure proper development of children and early detection of possible side effects.
- Advise clients to report signs and symptoms of fluid retention, throm-boembolic disorders, mental depression, or hepatic dysfunction to health-care professional.

ADMINISTRATION: IM, intranasal, subcutaneous, oral, IV, Depot or implant.

EVALUATION/DESIRED OUTCOME: Resolution of clinical symptoms of hormone imbalance including menopause symptoms and contraceptive; correction of fluid and electrolyte imbalances; control of the spread of advanced metastatic breast or prostate cancer; slowed progression of postmenopausal osteoporosis.

Laxatives

PURPOSE: Used to treat or prevent constipation or to prepare the bowel for radiologic or endoscopic procedures.

Type	Action	Example
Bulk-forming agents	Combine with water in the intestinal contents to form an emollient gel or viscous solution that promotes peristalsis and reduces transit time.	Polycarbophil (FiberCon®) Psyllium (Metamucil®)
Osmotics	Increase water content and softens the stool. May also be used for bowel prep for GI exam; Evacuation of the GI tract without electrolyte imbalance.	Polyethylene glycol/electrolyte (GoLYTELY®) Polyethylene glycol (MiraLax®) Phosphate/biphosphate (Fleet Enema®)
Magnesium	Used as treatment/prevention of hypomagnesium; essential for the activity of many enzymes.	Magnesium Citrate Magnesium Gluconate (Magtrate®) Magnesium Hydroxide (Phillips Milk of Magnesia®)
Stimulant laxatives	Stimulate peristalsis; alter fluid and electrolyte transport, producing fluid accumulation in the colon.	Bisacodyl (Dulcolax®) Sennosides (Senokot®)
Stool softeners	Promote incorporation of water in the stool, resulting in softer fecal mass.	Docusate (Surfak®)

Data Collection:
Baseline: vital signs, monitor for diarrhea; electrolytes, bowel patterns, serum sodium and phosphorus levels, serum calcium and potassium levels, acidosis; assess client for abdominal distention, presence of bowel sounds, and usual pattern of bowel function; assess color, consistency, and amount of stool produced; blood glucose levels; BUN levels.

Implementation:
- Excessive or prolonged use may lead to dependence.
- Laxatives may decrease the absorption of other orally administered drugs by decreasing transit time.
- Many laxatives may be administered at bedtime for morning results.
- Taking oral doses on an empty stomach will usually produce more rapid results.
- **Do not crush or chew enteric-coated tablets.** Take with a full glass of water or juice.
- Stool softeners and bulk laxatives may take several days for results.
- Advise clients, other than those with spinal cord injuries, that laxatives should be used only for short-term therapy.
- Advise client to increase fluid intake to a minimum of 1,500–2,000 mL/day during therapy to prevent dehydration.
- Encourage clients to use other forms of bowel regulation, such as increasing bulk in the diet, increasing fluid intake, and increasing mobility.
- Teach clients that normal bowel habits are individualized and may vary from three times per day to three times per week.
- Instruct clients with cardiac disease to avoid straining during bowel movements (Valsalva maneuver).
- Advise clients that laxatives should not be used when constipation is accompanied by abdominal pain, fever, nausea, or vomiting.

ADMINISTRATION: PO; available in powder, granules, or wafers; retention enema; oral solutions; sustained-release tablets; chewable tablets; rectal; granules, syrup, liquid.

EVALUATION/DESIRED OUTCOME: A soft, formed bowel movement; evacuation of the colon.

Lipid-Lowering Agents

PURPOSE: Used as a part of a total plan including diet and exercise to reduce blood lipids in an effort to reduce the morbidity and mortality of atherosclerotic cardiovascular disease and its sequelae.

Type	Action	Example
Bile acid sequestrants	Bind cholesterol in the GI tract forming an insoluble complex; result is increased clearance of cholesterol.	Cholestyramine (Questran®) Colesevelem (Welchol®) Colestipol (Colestid®)
HMG-CoA reductase inhibitors	Inhibit an enzyme involved in cholesterol synthesis.	Atorvastatin (Lipitor®) Pravastatin (Pravachol®) Rosuvastatin (Crestor®) Simvastatin (Zocor®)
Miscellaneous	Inhibits absorption of cholesterol in the intestine; inhibits triglyceride synthesis; inhibits peripheral lipolysis; increases HDL; large doses decrease lipoprotein and triglyceride synthesis.	Ezetimibe (Zetia®) Fenofibrate (TriCor®) Gemfibrozil (Lopid®) Niacin (Vitamin B)

Data Collection:
Baseline: serum total cholesterol, LDL, and triglyceride levels; prothrombin times; liver function tests (AST, ALT), phosphorus, chloride, and alkaline phosphatase, serum calcium, sodium, and potassium levels; monitor CPK levels, thyroid function tests; HgB, Hct, and WBCs, serum glucose.

Implementation:
■ Advise clients that these medications should be used in conjunction with diet restrictions (fat, cholesterol, carbohydrates, and alcohol), exercise, and cessation of smoking.

ADMINISTRATION: PO, powder for suspension with aspartame, powder for suspension, unflavored; granules for suspension, flavored granules for suspension; IV.

EVALUATION/DESIRED OUTCOME: Decreased serum triglyceride and LDL cholesterol levels and improved HDL cholesterol ratios. Therapy is usually discontinued if the clinical response is not evident after 3 months of therapy.

Nonopioid Analgesics

PURPOSE: Used to control mild to moderate pain, fever, or both. Phenazopyridine is used to treat urinary tract pain, and capsaicin is used topically for a variety of painful syndromes.

Type	Action	Example
Nonsteroidal anti-inflammatory agents	Inhibit prostaglandin synthesis.	Diclofenac (Voltaren®) Etodolac (Lodine XL®) Ibuprofen (Advil®, Motrin®) Ketorolac (Toradol®) Valdecoxib (Bextra®)
Salicylates	Produce analgesia and reduce inflammation and fever by inhibiting the production of prostaglandins. Aspirin decreases platelet aggregation.	Aspirin Choline and magnesium salicylates (Trilisate®) Choline salicylate (Arthropan®) Magnesium salicylate (Doan's Regular Strength Tablets®)
Miscellaneous	Inhibit the synthesis of prostaglandins that may serve as mediators of pain and fever, primarily in the CNS.	Acetaminophen (Tylenol®) Butalbital compounds (Fiorinal®) Capsaicin (Zostrix®) Naproxen sodium (Aleve®)

Data Collection:

Baseline: Hgb, Hct, leukocyte, and platelet counts; liver function tests; BUN, serum creatinine, and electrolytes, decreased urine electrolyte concentrations, blood glucose, prolonged bleeding time; serum potassium, urine albumin, bilirubin, 17-ketosteroid, 17-hydroxycorticosteriod; interferes with urine tests based on color reactions (glucose, ketones, bilirubin, steroids, protein); plasma amylase; lipase concentration; may alter urine 5-HIAA and urine steroid determination.

Implementation:

■ Instruct clients to take salicylates and NSAIDs with a full glass of water and to remain in an upright position for 15–30 min after administration.

■ Adults should not take acetaminophen longer than 10 days and children not longer than 5 days unless directed by a health-care professional.

■ Short-term doses of acetaminophen with salicylates or NSAIDs should not exceed the recommended daily dose of either drug alone.

■ Caution clients to avoid concurrent use of alcohol with this medication to minimize gastric irritation.

■ Caution clients to avoid taking acetaminophen, salicylates, or NSAIDs concurrently for more than a few days, unless directed by health-care professional, to prevent analgesic neuropathy.

■ Advise clients undergoing long-term therapy to inform health-care professionals of medication regimen prior to surgery.

ADMINISTRATION: PO, topical; administer after meals, with food, or with an antacid containing aluminum or magnesium to minimize gastric irritation; do not crush, break, or chew extended release tablets; IM; IV; topical.

EVALUATION/DESIRED OUTCOME: Relief of mild to moderate discomfort; reduction of fever.

Nonsteroidal Anti-Inflammatory Agents

PURPOSE: NSAIDs are used to control mild to moderate pain, fever, and various inflammatory conditions, such as rheumatoid arthritis and osteoarthritis. Ophthalmic NSAIDs are used to decrease postoperative ocular inflammation, to inhibit perioperative miosis, and to decrease inflammation from allergies.

Type	Action	Example
Nonsteroidal anti-inflammatory agents	Analgesic and anti-inflammatory effects result from inhibition of prostaglandin synthesis. Antipyretic action results from vasodilatation and inhibition of prostaglandin synthesis in the CNS.	Celecoxib (Celebrex®) Diclofenac (Voltaren®) Ibuprofen (Advil®) Indomethacin (Indocin®) Ketorolac (Toradol®) Nabumetone (Relafen®) Naproxen (Aleve®)
Ophthalmic NSAIDs		Diclofenac (Voltaren®) Flurbiprofen (Oculen®) Ketorolac (Acular®) Suprofen (Profenal®)

Data Collection:
Baseline: vital signs; AST and ALT levels; phosphate levels; BUN; creatinine and electrolytes: hemoglobin, hematocrit, leukocyte, and platelet counts; serum alkaline phosphatase, LDH; urine uric acid concentrations; blood glucose; urine albumin, bilirubin, 17-ketosteroid, and 17-hydroxycorticosteroid determinations; may cause prolonged bleeding.

Implementation:
■ Caution clients not to wear hydrocel contact lenses concurrently while taking ophthalmic NSAIDs.

■ Administer NSAIDs after meals or with food or an antacid to minimize gastric irritation.

■ Instruct clients to take NSAIDs with a full glass of water and to remain in an upright position for 15–30 min after administration.

- Caution clients to avoid concurrent use of alcohol with this medication to minimize possible gastric irritation.
- Caution clients to avoid taking acetaminophen, salicylates, or NSAIDs concurrently for more than a few days, unless directed by health-care professional, to prevent analgesic nephropathy.
- Advise clients undergoing long-term therapy to inform health-care professional of medication regimen prior to surgery.

ADMINISTRATION: Capsules; PO, topical; IM, IV.

EVALUATION/DESIRED OUTCOME: Relief of mild to moderate discomfort; reduction of fever.

Opioid Analgesics

PURPOSE: Management of moderate to severe pain.

Type	Action	Example
Opioid agonists/ antagonists	Bind to opiate receptors in the CNS; Alters the perception of and response to painful stimuli while producing generalized CNS depression.	Buprenorphine (Buprenex®) Butorphanol (Stadol®) Pentazocine (Talwin®)
Opioid agonists	Bind to opiate receptors in the CNS, altering response to and perception of pain.	Codeine Fentanyl Fentanyl (Transdermal) (Duragesic®) Hydrocodone (Hycodan®) Hydromorphone (Dilaudid®) Meperidine (Demerol®) Methadone (Dolophine®) Morphine (Duramorph®) Oxycodone (OxyContin®)

Baseline: vital signs; serum amylase and lipase levels, liver function tests, AST, ALT, serum alkaline phosphatase, LDH, and bilirubin concentrations.

Implementation:

- Do not confuse morphine with hydromorphone or meperidine; errors have resulted in fatalities.
- Explain therapeutic value of medication before administration to enhance the analgesic effect.
- Regularly administered doses may be more effective than prn administration. Analgesic is more effective if given before pain becomes severe.
- Coadministration with nonopioid analgesics may have additive analgesic effects and may permit lower doses.
- Medication should be discontinued gradually after long-term use to prevent withdrawal.
- Instruct clients on how and when to ask for pain medication.
- Medication may cause drowsiness or dizziness.
- Advise clients to make position changes slowly to minimize orthostatic hypotension.
- Caution clients to avoid concurrent use of alcohol or other CNS depressants with this medication.
- Encourage clients to turn, cough, and breathe deeply every 2 hours to prevent atelectasis.

ADMINISTRATION: IM, IV, sublingual, intranasal; transmucosal; transdermal; oral elixir solution; subcu; rectal; epidural.

EVALUATION/DESIRED OUTCOME: Decreased severity of pain without a significant alteration in level of consciousness or respiratory status.

Sedative/Hypnotics

PURPOSE: Sedatives are used to provide sedation, usually prior to procedures. Hypnotics are used to manage insomnia.

Type	Action	Example
Barbiturates	Used to treat seizures	Phenobarbital
Benzodiazepines	Act at many levels of the CNS to produce anxiolytic effect; effects may be mediated by GABA, an inhibitory neurotransmitter.	Chlordiazepoxide (Librium®) Diazepam (Valium®) Flurazepam (Dalmane®) Lorazepam (Ativan®) Midazolam (Versed®) Triazolam (Halcion®)
Miscellaneous	Alter the action of dopamine in the CNS.	Droperidol (Inapsine®) Promethazine (Phenergan®) Hydroxyzine (Atarax®) Zolpidem (Ambien®)

Data Collection:
Baseline: vital signs; CBC and liver function tests, bilirubin, AST, ALT; urine 17-ketosteroids, 17-ketogenic steroids; urinary catecholamines; thyroidal uptake; hepatic and renal function tests; may cause false-negative results in skin tests using allergen extracts; may cause false-positive pregnancy test results; serum glucose; EKG.

Implementation:
- Supervise ambulation and transfer of clients following administration of hypnotic doses.
- Remove cigarettes.
- Raise side rails and ensure that call bell is within reach at all times.
- Keep bed in low position.
- Discuss with clients the importance of preparing the environment for sleep. If medication is less effective after a few weeks, advise clients to consult health-care professionals; do not increase dose.
- Gradual withdrawal may be required to prevent reactions following prolonged therapy.

- Sedatives/hypnotics may cause daytime drowsiness. Caution clients to avoid driving and other activities requiring alertness until response to medication is known.
- Advise clients to avoid the use of alcohol and other CNS depressants concurrently with these medications.
- Advise clients to inform health-care professional if pregnancy is planned or suspected.

ADMINISTRATION: PO, IM, IV, rectal.

EVALUATION/DESIRED OUTCOME: Improvement in sleep patterns; control of seizures; decrease in muscle spasms; decreased tremulousness; more rational ideation when used for alcohol withdrawal.

Controlled Substances		
Schedule I	High potential for abuse; **No accepted medical use in US**	Heroin, LSD, marijuana
Schedule II	High potential for abuse; **Used in US with severe restrictions**	Morphine, cocaine, methadone, methamphetamine
Schedule III	Potential for low or moderate physical dependence or high psychological dependence; used in United States as medical treatment	Anabolic steroids, codeine, hydrocodone, some barbiturates
Schedule IV	Low potential for abuse; used in United States as medical treatment	Darvon®, Talwin®, Valium®, Xanax®
Schedule V	Low potential for abuse; used in United States as medical treatment	Over-the-counter cough syrup with codeine

Source: U.S. Department of Justice, Drug Enforcement Administration, Initial Schedule of Controlled Substances. Available at: http://www.usdoj.gov/dea/pubs/csa/812.htm#c.

Skeletal Muscle Relaxants

PURPOSE: Two major uses are spasticity associated with spinal cord diseases or lesions or adjunctive therapy in the symptomatic relief of acute painful musculoskeletal conditions. Also may be used to treat and prevent malignant hyperthermia.

Type	Action	Example
Centrally acting	Depress the CNS, probably by potentiating GABA, an inhibitory neurotransmitter; produce skeletal muscle by inhibiting spinal polysynaptic afferent pathways.	Diazepam (Valium®) Orphenadrine (Norflex®) Baclofen (Lioresal®) Cyclobenzaprine (Flexeril®) Methocarbamol (Robaxin®)
Direct acting		Dantrolene (Dantrium®)

Data Collection:
Baseline: vital signs; hepatic and renal function, CBC; serum glucose, alkaline phosphatase, AST, and ALT levels; may cause false-positive Benedict's test results; may cause falsely increased urinary 5-hydroxyindoleacetic acid (5-HIAA) and vanillylmandelic (VMA) determinations; serum bilirubin.

Implementation:
- Provide safety measures as indicated.
- Supervise ambulation and transfer of clients.
- Encourage clients to comply with additional therapies prescribed for muscle spasm (rest, physical therapy, heat).
- Medication may cause drowsiness. Caution clients to avoid driving or other activities requiring mental alertness until response to drug is known.
- Advise clients to avoid concurrent use of alcohol or other CNS depressants with these medications.

ADMINISTRATION: PO, IV, IM; test dose and titration; intermittent infusion.

Vascular Headache Suppressants

PURPOSE: Used for acute treatment of vascular headaches (migraine, cluster headaches, and migraine variants). Other agents such as some beta blockers and some calcium channel blockers are used for suppression of frequently occurring vascular headaches.

Type	Action	Example
Alpha-adrenergic blockers	In therapeutic doses, produce vasoconstriction of dilated blood vessels by stimulating alpha-adrenergic and serotonergic (5-HT) receptors.	Dihydroergotamine (Migranal®) Ergotamine (Ergostat®)
Beta-blockers	Block stimulation of beta$_1$ (myocardial) and beta$_2$ (pulmonary, vascular, and uterine) adrenergic receptor sites.	Propranolol (Inderal®) Timilol (Blocadren®)
5-HT, agonists	Act as an agonist at specific 5-HT, receptor sites in intracranial blood vessels and sensory trigeminal nerve ending.	Almotriptan (Axert®) Eletriptan (Relpax®) Sumatriptan (Imitrex®)
Miscellaneous	Increase levels of GABA, an inhibitory transmitter in the CNS; inhibit the transport of calcium into myocardial and vascular smooth muscle cells resulting in inhibition of excitation-contraction coupling and subsequent contraction.	Divalproex sodium (Depakote®) Valproate sodium (Depacon®) Valproic acid (Depakene®) Verapamil (Calan®)

Data Collection:

Baseline: vital signs, EKG monitoring, pulmonary capillary wedge pressure (PCWP), central venous pressure (CVP), intake and output ratios, daily weights; assess for signs of fluid overload (peripheral edema, dyspnea, rales/crackles, fatigue, weight gain, jugular venous distention); BUN, serum lipoprotein, potassium, triglyceride, and uric acid levels; ANA titers, blood glucose levels; hepatic and renal levels; thyroid function tests; may cause false-positive results in urine ketone tests; total serum calcium concentrations; serum potassium levels.

Implementation:

- Medication should be administered at the first sign of a headache.
- Inform clients that medication should be used only during a migraine attack. It is meant to be used for relief of migraine attacks but not to prevent or reduce the number of attacks.
- Advise clients that lying down in a darkened room following medication administration may further help relieve headache.
- May cause dizziness or drowsiness. Caution client to avoid driving or other activities requiring alertness until response to medication is known.
- Advise clients to avoid alcohol, which aggravates headaches.

ADMINISTRATION: PO, SL, intranasal, IM, subcu, IV, intermittent infusions.

EVALUATION/DESIRED OUTCOME: Relief of migraine attack.

Educating Clients About Safe Medication Use

- **Generic and brand names of the medication:** Clients should know both the brand and the generic names of each medication.
- **Purpose of the medication:** Clients should understand the therapeutic benefits of their medications and should understand the possible consequences of failing to take their medications as prescribed.
- **Dosage and how to take the medication:** Clients must know how much of the medication to take and when to take it.
- **What to do if a dose is missed:** Clients sometimes take a double dose of medications when a missed dose occurs, putting themselves at risk for side effects and adverse reactions.

- **Duration of therapy**: Instruct clients regarding the importance of continuing a medication even when they feel better or when they cannot perceive a benefit.
- **Minor side effects and what to do if they occur**: Inform clients that all medications have potential side effects. Explain the most common side effects associated with the medication and how to avoid or manage them if they occur.
- **Serious side effects and what to do if they occur**: Describe signs and symptoms associated with serious side effects and tell clients to immediately inform a physician or nurse if they occur.
- **Medications to avoid**: Advise clients (and family if needed) as to which medications, including which over-the-counter medications, to avoid.
- **Food–drug interactions**: Instruct clients that such interactions are not uncommon and can have effects similar to drug–drug interactions.
- **How to store the medication**: Instruct clients on proper storage of medications to maintain potency.
- **Follow-up care**: Advise clients regarding the importance of ongoing care to assess effectiveness and appropriateness of medications.
- **What not to take**: Inform clients not to take expired medications or someone else's medication.

Medical/Surgical Nursing

Acid–Base Imbalances

Body's Response to Acid–Base Imbalance				
	pH	HCO₃	pCO₂	Compensation
Respiratory acidosis	↓	↑ or normal	↑	Kidneys conserve HCO₃ and eliminate H⁺ to ↑ pH.
Respiratory alkalosis	↑	↓ or normal	↓	Kidneys eliminate HCO₃ and conserve H⁺ to ↓ pH.
Metabolic acidosis	↓	↓	↓ or normal	Hyperventilation blows off excess CO₂ and conserves HCO₃.
Metabolic alkalosis	↑	↑	↑ or normal	Hypoventilation to ↑ CO₂. Kidneys retain H⁺ and excrete HCO₃.

Respiratory Acidosis

■ **Causes:** Caused by respiratory problems; acute respiratory acidosis is caused by hypoventilation from drugs or neurological problems that depress breathing.

■ **Signs/Symptoms:** Confusion progressing to lethargy to stupor and coma if not treated; shortness of breath, fatigue, sleepiness.

■ **Treatment:** Aggressive management of underlying respiratory problem.

Respiratory Alkalosis

■ **Causes:** Caused by hyperventilation resulting from prolonged mechanical ventilation, high altitudes, and excessive fear and anxiety and during pulmonary examination.

■ **Signs/Symptoms:** Serum pH increases; light-headedness, dizziness, numbness of hands and feet, heart rate increases, pulse is weak and thready.

■ **Treatment:** Have client hold breath or rebreathe own carbon dioxide with the use of a paper bag or a rebreather mask; underlying cause also must be treated.

- **Causes:** Overuse or abuse of antacids or baking soda, prolonged vomiting, or nasogastric suctioning.
- **Signs/Symptoms** Related to hypokalemia (weakness, dysrhythmias) and hypocalcemia (headache, lethargy, neuromuscular excitability).
- **Treatment:** Identify the underlying cause and manage it as quickly as possible.

Metabolic Acidosis

- **Causes:** Caused by too much acid in the body or too little bicarbonate in the body; common causes are uncontrolled diabetes mellitus, end-stage renal failure, severe diarrhea, or prolonged nasogastric suction.
- **Signs/Symptoms:** Serum pH decreases as the bicarbonate level decreases; confusion, lethargy, Kussmaul respirations.
- **Treatment:** Aggressive management of underlying respiratory problem.

Adult Vital Signs

Normal Adult Vital Signs

Heart Rate	Respiratory Rate	Systolic Blood Pressure (top number)	Diastolic Blood Pressure (bottom number)
60–100 beats/min	12–20 breaths/min	95–140 mmHg	60–90 mmHg

Temperature		
Tympanic	98.6°F–100.6°F	37.0°C–38.1°C
Axillary	96.6°F–100.6°F	35.9°C–37.0°C
Oral	97.6°F–99.6°F	36.4°C–37.6°C
Rectal	98.6°F–100.6°F	37.0°C–38.1°C

- Obtain client's vital signs per facility protocol or physician order.
- NEVER take a blood pressure on an arm with a dialysis shunt, injury, or same side mastectomy or axillary surgery.
- **Increased heart rate can be caused by:** fever, anxiety, acute pain, cardiac tamponade, congestive heart failure (CHF), pulmonary embolism, exercise, decreased hemoglobin and hematocrit, abnormal blood sugar, decreased potassium, and abnormal sodium levels.
- **Increased temperature can be caused by:** fever, CHF, pulmonary embolism, and exercise.
- **Increased blood pressure can be caused by:** anxiety, pain, exercise, increased sodium, and increased potassium levels.
- Document the time and client vital signs.
- Document temperature reading and route.
- Report abnormal values to team leader or RN.

Cardiopulmonary Resuscitation (CPR)

Determine unresponsiveness.

- Call 911; get help; obtain automated external defibrillator (AED) if available.
- Infant or child: Call 911 after 2 minutes (five cycles) of CPR.

Airway: Open the airway.

- Tilt head; lift chin.
- Use jaw thrust method if necessary.

Breathing: Assess for breathing.

- If not breathing, give two slow breaths at 1 second per breath.
- If unsuccessful, reposition airway and reattempt ventilation.
- If still unsuccessful, refer to Choking section.

Circulation: Check for a pulse for 10 seconds.

- Adult or child: Check carotid artery.
- Infant: Check brachial or femoral artery.
- If pulse is present but client is not breathing, begin rescue breathing.
- Adult: 10–12 breaths/min.

- Child or infant: 12–20 breaths/min.
- Newborn: 40–60 breaths/min.
- If no pulse after 10 seconds, begin chest compressions.

Automated external defibrillator (AED): Power on and follow commands.

- Perform 2 minutes of CPR between each shock.
- Do not use pediatric pads on adults.
- Infant or child: Use after 2 minutes (five cycles) of CPR.
- Recheck pulse every 5 minutes and after each shock.

	Adult	Child/Infant	Newborn
Ventilation rate	10–12/min	12–20/min	40–60/min
Compression rate	100/min	100/min	120/min
Ratio	30:2 (1 or 2 rescuers)	30:2 (1 rescuer) 15:2 (2 rescuers)	3:1 (1 or 2 rescuers)
Compression depth	1.5–2 inches	½ to ⅓ the depth of the chest	⅓ the depth of the chest

CPR Maneuvers

Head-Tilt, Chin-Lift: Adult/Child

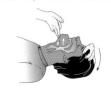

Jaw-Thrust: Adult/Child
For known or suspected trauma

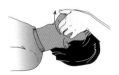

Pulse Check: Adult/Child (Carotid)

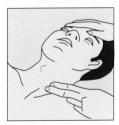

Pulse Check: Infant (Brachial)

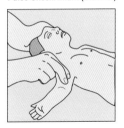

Hand Placement: Adult/Child
Lower half of sternum

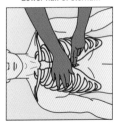

Finger Placement: Infant
One finger width below nipples

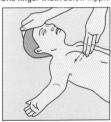

Choking

Conscious Victim

Assess for airway obstruction.

- Adult or child: if choking, look for universal choking sign (both hands grasping neck); check for ability to speak.
- Infant: Check for inability to cry or ineffective cry.

Attempt to relieve obstruction.

- Adult or child: Perform Heimlich maneuver until the obstruction is removed or victim becomes unresponsive.
- Infant: Give five back blows and five chest thrusts until the obstruction is removed or infant becomes unresponsive.

Unresponsive Victim

Determine unresponsiveness.

- Adult: Call 911 before any intervention.
- Infant or child: Call 911 after 1 minute of attempting to remove obstruction.

Open airway.

- Place victim in supine position in a safe area.
- Tilt head; lift chin.
- Use jaw thrust method if necessary.

Assess breathing and attempt to ventilate.

- Adult or child: Straddle victim's thighs and perform abdominal thrusts.
- Infants: Give five back blows and five chest compressions.

Inspect mouth and remove obstruction.

- Adult: Lift jaw and tongue; sweep mouth.
- Infant or child: Lift jaw and tongue; remove obstruction only if seen. DO NOT sweep mouth.

Repeat the following steps until obstruction is removed:

1. Inspect
2. Sweep (if applicable)
3. Ventilate
4. Perform abdominal blows or back thrusts

Note: If victim begins breathing, place in recovery position and recheck ABCs (airway, breathing, circulation) every minute.

Heimlich Maneuver

Hemlich Maneuver: Adult/Child
Use chest thrusts for head/neck

**Hemlich Maneuver:
Unresponsive Adult/Child**
Stay well below the xyphoid

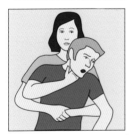 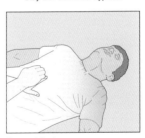

Back blows and chest thrusts: Infant
Always support head/neck

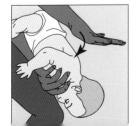 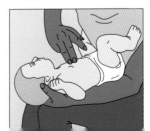

Recovery Position
Reassess ABCs frequently

Head-tilt, Chin-Lift: Infant
Do not hyperextent the neck

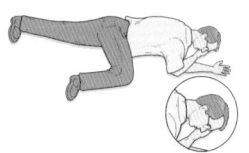 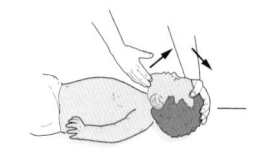

Recovery Position

Fluid and Electrolyte Imbalances

Fluid Volume Deficit
- **Causes:** NPO status; hemorrhage; sweating; diuretic therapy; diarrhea; vomiting; GI suctioning; draining fistulas, wounds, and abscesses; systemic infection; fever; enemas; ileostomy; cecostomy; diabetes insipidus.
- **Signs/Symptoms:** Thirst; poor skin turgor; elevated temperature; urine output decreased; constipation; weight loss; decreased blood pressure.
- **Associated Lab Data:** Urine output less than 30 mL/hour; elevated hematocrit; elevated BUN; increased urinary specific gravity.

Fluid Volume Excess
- **Causes:** Too much fluid in bloodstream; dilution of electrolytes and red blood cells.
- **Signs/Symptoms:** Increased blood pressure; bounding pulse; increased, shallow respirations; pitting edema in feet and legs; pale, cool skin; increased urine output; increased weight gain; dyspnea; excess peritoneal fluid; moist crackles in the lungs.
- **Associated Lab Data:** Decreased BUN; decreased hematocrit; decreased urinary specific gravity

Nursing Interventions for Fluid Volume Deficit and Excess

- Monitor weight loss or weight gain.
- If IV therapy is used, monitor isotonic fluid replacement for dehydration.
- For clients with fluid excess, use an electronic infusion pump or a burette to control the rate of infusion.
- Weigh client before breakfast at the same time each day with the same amount of clothing and using the same scale.
- For clients in their homes, they should be weighed at least three times per week.
- For clients in nursing homes, on admission, they should be weighed once a week for 4 weeks; then once a month.
- Intake and output should be recorded daily.
- Offer fluids to clients with cognitive impairment, if dehydration is present.
- Monitor for fluid excess, especially if IV fluids are being given.
- Teach client and family members to report early signs and symptoms of dehydration or fluid excess.
- If overhydration is present, place client in semi-Fowler's or high-Fowler's position.
- If ordered, place client on oxygen infusing no higher that 2 L/min.
- Administer diuretic if ordered. Monitor strict intake and output if diuretics are ordered.
- Report if urinary output falls below 30 mL/hour to the physician or the RN.

Hypercalcemia (Calcium Excess)

- **Causes:** Excessive intake of calcium or vitamin D; renal failure; hyperparathyroidism, invasive or metastatic cancers; overuse or prolonged use of thiazide diuretics.
- **Signs/Symptoms:** Increased heart rate and blood pressure; skeletal muscle weakness; decreased GI motility; decreased blood clotting capability; renal calculi; urinary calculi; respiratory failure; heart failure.
- **Associated Lab Data:** Serum calcium higher than 11 mg/dL or 5.5 mEq/L; abnormal ECG.

Hypocalcemia (Calcium Deficit)

- **Causes:** Occurs slowly as a result of chronic disease or poor intake; postmenopausal; inadequate absorption of calcium from the intestines, such as in Crohn's disease; partial or complete surgical removal of the thyroid or parathyroid; renal failure resulting in hyperphosphatemia.
- **Signs/Symptoms:** Increased and irregular heart rate; mental status changes; hyperactive deep tendon reflexes; increased GI motility, including diarrhea and abdominal cramping; seizures; respiratory failure; cardiac failure.
- **Associated Lab Data:** Serum calcium less than 9 mg/dL or 4.5 mEq/L; abnormal ECG; increased parathyroid hormone.

Nursing Interventions for Hypercalcemia and hypocalcemia

- Instruct clients with low calcium levels to take calcium supplements 1 to 2 hours after meals to increase intestinal absorption.
- If client has had thyroid or parathyroid surgery, have calcium gluconate or calcium chloride next to the bedside for emergency use.
- For clients with renal failure and hyperphosphatemia, the physician may order aluminum hydroxide to bind excess phosphate in the GI tract. Monitor both phosphate and calcium levels.
- Teach client and family about increasing calcium-enriched foods in diet if the client's calcium level is low.
- Teach client and family about increasing vitamin D intake to help with calcium absorption.
- Teach clients about the proper amount of calcium needed each day and the dangers of taking in too much calcium.
- If clients have excess calcium, they should be hospitalized and placed on cardiac monitoring.
- If ordered, start IV and infuse normal saline to promote renal excretion of calcium. Monitor intake and output.
- Instruct that the physician may discontinue thiazide diuretics and prescribe diuretics that promote calcium excretion.
- Teach client and family members about other drugs that may be used to increase calcium excretion.
- Monitor the client's calcium level if placed on hemodialysis, peritoneal dialysis, or ultrafiltration to remove calcium.

Hyperkalemia (Potassium excess)

- **Causes:** Overuse of potassium-based salt substitutes; excessive intake of oral or IV potassium; use of potassium-sparing diuretics; renal failure; massive trauma.
- **Signs/Symptoms:** Muscle cramping can occur with either potassium deficit or excess; muscular weakness; increased GI motility (diarrhea); slow, irregular heart rate; decreased blood pressure.
- **Associated Lab Data:** Serum potassium level exceeds 5 mEq/L.; ECG may show irregularities; metabolic acidosis may be present; serum pH falls below 7.35.

Hypokalemia (Potassium Deficit)

- **Causes:** Inadequate intake of potassium; excessive loss of potassium through the kidneys; losses through medication; excessive diarrhea; severe vomiting; prolonged GI suction; major surgery and hemorrhage.
- **Signs/Symptoms:** Muscle cramping; shallow, ineffective respirations; pulse is weak, irregular, and thready; possible irregular heartbeats; orthostatic hypotension; GI motility slowed (constipation).
- **Associated Lab Data:** Serum potassium level falls below 3.5 mEq/L.
- ECG may show irregularities; metabolic alkalosis may be present; serum pH higher than 7.45.

Nursing Interventions for Hyperkalemia and Hypokalemia

- Administer oral potassium supplements, if ordered, to increase potassium levels.
- If IV potassium is used to correct hypokalemia, make sure the client has voided before administering IV fluids with potassium.
- Double-check the label on the IV fluids to ensure accuracy.
- **Never give potassium IV push.**
- **Administration of IV potassium is the responsibility of the RN.**
- Teach client and family not to substitute one potassium supplement for another.
- Dilute powders and liquids according to manufacturer's recommendations.
- Teach client not to drink diluted solutions until the oral potassium is thoroughly mixed.
- Do not crush potassium tablets. Check with manufacturer's directions regarding whether the tablets can be crushed.
- Administer slow-release tablets with 8 oz of water.

- Instruct client to avoid taking potassium supplements if taking a potassium-sparing diuretic.
- Instruct client not to use salt substitutes containing potassium unless prescribed by the physician.
- Instruct to take potassium with meals.
- Tell client which adverse effects need to be reported to the health-care professional.
- Instruct on the importance of monitoring potassium levels.
- If potassium excess is present, teach the client to avoid high potassium foods (i.e., bananas).
- Monitor the client if the physician orders potassium-losing diuretics.
- If the client has renal disease, the physician may order Kayexalate® either orally or rectally. Monitor the serum potassium level.
- Monitor cardiac telemetry.

Hypermagnesemia (Magnesium Excess)
- **Causes:** Increased intake; decreased renal excretion caused by renal failure.
- **Signs/Symptoms:** Symptoms usually are not present until level is 4 mEq/L; bradycardia; dysrhythmias; hypotension; lethargy or drowsiness; skeletal muscle weakness; coma, respiratory or cardiac failure can occur if not treated.
- **Associated Lab Data:** Serum magnesium level increases to 2.5 mEq/L or greater.

Hypomagnesemia (Magnesium Deficit)
- **Causes:** Decreased intake from malnutrition and starvation diets; Crohn's disease; alcoholism; loop and osmotic diuretics; certain antibiotics; some anticancer agents.
- **Signs/Symptoms:** Imbalance of magnesium usually accompanied by imbalance of calcium; signs and symptoms are similar to hypocalcemia.
- **Associated Lab Data:** Serum magnesium level falls below 1.5 mEq/L.

Nursing Interventions for Hypermagnesemia and Hypomagnesemia

- Monitor client's vital signs if client receives magnesium IV to increase the magnesium level.
- If calcium level is low, administer calcium replacements as ordered by physician.
- Place client on cardiac monitoring.
- Have emergency medications available if client experiences life-threatening dysrhythmias.
- If client has good kidney functioning, loop diuretics can be used to flush out the excess magnesium.
- Monitor IV fluids if used to flush out the excess magnesium.
- If the client has inadequate renal function, dialysis may be the only option.

Hypernatremia (Sodium Excess)

- **Causes:** Too much sodium; inability to excrete the sodium, such as in renal failure.
- **Signs/Symptoms:** Thirst; may have mental status changes, such as agitation, confusion, and personality changes; seizures may occur; muscle twitches and contractions; skeletal muscles weaken leading to respiratory arrest.
- **Associated Lab Data:** Serum sodium level is higher than 145 mEq/L; increased sodium osmolarity; increased BUN; elevated hematocrit; increased urinary specific gravity.

Hyponatremia (Sodium Deficit)

- **Causes:** Inadequate intake of sodium; excessive sodium loss from the body; plasma volume increases causing delusional effect; high fever; strenuous exercise or physical labor.
- **Signs/Symptoms:** Decreased sodium usually is accompanied by fluid imbalance resulting in dehydration; decreased sodium with fluid excess results in overhydration; disorientation; confusion; and personality changes; weakness, nausea, vomiting, and diarrhea; if severe enough, respiratory arrest and coma can occur.
- **Associated Lab Data:** Serum sodium level less than 135 mEq/L; decreased serum chloride.

Nursing Interventions for Hypernatremia and Hyponatremia

- If ordered, start an IV of normal saline for clients who have decreased sodium without fluid excess.
- If client has fluid excess and decreased sodium, fluid restriction may be ordered.
- If ordered, administer diuretic, or steroids, if cerebral edema is present.
- Strict monitoring of intake and output (I&O).
- Weigh client daily.
- If ordered, start an IV of 5% dextrose in water to correct sodium excess.
- If kidneys are functioning, diuretics may be used to rid the body of excess sodium.
- If kidneys are not functioning, dialysis may be ordered.
- If a sodium-restricted diet is ordered, teach client and family members about foods to be avoided (i.e., dietary products, grain products, salted and processed foods).

Pain

Pain experience differs between and among individuals of differing cultural, ethnic, or religious groups.

Types of Pain

- Acute.
- Cancer related.
- Chronic nonmalignant.

Treatment of Pain

- Three classes of analgesics: opioids, nonopioids, and adjuvants.
- Radiation therapy.
- Antineoplastic chemotherapy.
- Placebos.
- Nondrug therapies: Cognitive–behavioral interventions and physical agents (heat or cold, massage, exercise, immobilization, and transcutaneous electrical nerve stimulation [TENS])

World Health Organization Analgesic Ladder

Helps direct the interventions required when using medications to treat cancer pain and other types of pain.

- **Level I:** Clients are experiencing mild pain; nonopioid analgesics are used to control the pain.
- **Level II:** Clients are experiencing mild to moderate pain; opioids are added to the nonopioids.
- **Level III:** Clients are experiencing moderate to severe pain; adjuvant analgesics are added to the nonopioid and opioid analgesics.

Nursing Interventions
- Assess pain based on what the client says.
- Assess the client's pain using a pain rating scale. Use the same scale consistently.
- Assess whether pain is acute, chronic, or both.

- Assess if client needs emotional or spiritual support.
- Following World Health Organization's pain management ladder, give analgesics before pain becomes severe.
- Combine opioid and nonopioid analgesics as ordered.
- Assess pain relief approximately 1 hour after administration of oral analgesics or 30 minutes after IV analgesic.
- Observe for anticipated adverse effects of pain medication.
- If opioids are being used, assess for respiratory depression and level of sedation at regular intervals.
- Prevent constipation by encouraging the client to drink 8 to 10 glasses of fluid daily, eat more foods with fiber, take fiber or bulk laxatives, and exercise as tolerated.
- Teach client nondrug pain relief interventions, such as relaxation and distraction, to be used with the medications.

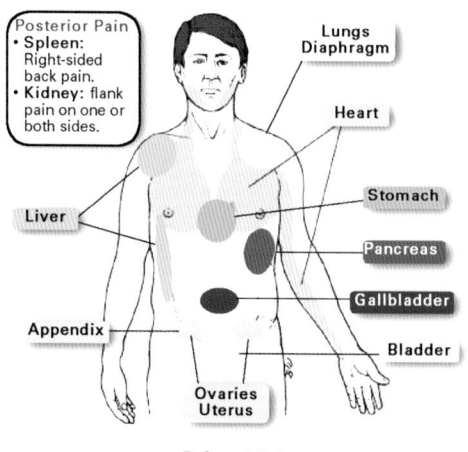

Referred Pain

Numeric Pain Scale

0	1	2	3	4	5	6	7	8	9	10
No pain										Worst pain

	Mild		Moderate			Severe

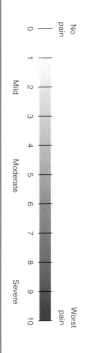

Wong-Baker FACES Pain Rating Scale

0	2	4	6	8	10
NO HURT	HURTS LITTLE BIT	HURTS LITTLE MORE	HURTS EVEN MORE	HURTS WHOLE LOT	HURTS WORST

Source: Hockenberry, MJ, Wilson D, Winkelstein ML. *Wong's Essentials of Pediatric Nursing*, ed 7, St. Louis, 2005, p. 1259. Used with permission. Copyright Mosby.

Shock

Hypovolemic Shock

- **Causes:** Dehydration; internal or external hemorrhage; fluid loss from burns; vomiting or diarrhea; loss of intravascular fluid as a result of sepsis or trauma.
- **Symptoms:** Pale, cool, clammy skin; tachycardia; tachypnea; flat, nondistended peripheral veins; decreased jugular vein; decreased urine output; and altered mental status.

Cardiogenic Shock

- **Causes:** Heart fails to pump; acute myocardial infarction; 40% of myocardium must be lost to produce cardiogenic shock; rupture of heart valves; acute myocarditis; end-stage heart disease; severe dysrhythmias; traumatic injury to the heart.
- **Symptoms:** Distended jugular and peripheral veins, symptoms of heart failure, pulmonary edema. Presence of pulmonary edema differentiates cardiogenic shock from other shocks.

Obstructive Shock

- **Causes:** Pericardial tamponade; tension pneumothorax; acute pulmonary hypertension; tumors or large emboli.
- **Symptoms:** Symptoms similar to hypovolemic shock except that jugular veins are usually distended.

Distributive Shock

- **Causes:** Anaphylactic shock occurs when the body has an extreme hypersensitivity reaction to an antigen, such as insect stings, antibiotics, shellfish, peanuts, anesthetics, contrast dye, and blood products. Septic shock is caused by systemic infection and inflammation; neurogenic shock occurs when dysfunction or injury to the nervous system causes excessive distention of peripheral blood vessels.

- **Symptoms:** Anaphylactic shock: signs and symptoms are similar to hypovolemic shock, urticaria, pruritis, wheezing, laryngeal edema, angioedema, and severe bronchospasm.
- During the early phase of septic shock, blood pressure, urine output, and neck vein size may be normal; fever may be present. Second phase symptoms include hypotension, oliguria, tachycardia, tachypnea, flat jugular and peripheral veins, and cold, clammy skin; body temperature may be normal or subnormal.

Diagnostic Tests for Shock

- **Laboratory Tests:** Complete blood count (CBC), serum osmolarity, blood chemistries, prothrombin time, partial thromboplastin time, blood typing and cross match, serum lactate, arterial blood gases, cardiac isoenzymes, urinalysis.
- **Imaging:** Chest x-ray, spinal films, computed tomography, echocardiogram.
- **Monitoring:** Electrocardiogram; arterial pressure monitor; central venous pressure; pulmonary artery catheter, gastric pH.

Nursing Interventions for Shock

- Maintain airway and provide oxygenation.
- Monitor vital signs.
- Monitor intake and output.
- Provide adequate fluid intake.
- Position client appropriately (head elevated for clients with shortness of breath or increased intracranial pressure).
- Provide quiet, restful environment.
- Maintain body temperature with warmed IV fluids, room temperature, and blankets.
- Assess for pain and provide pain relief measures.
- Change position slowly to prevent orthostatic hypotension.
- Monitor heart rate and cardiac rhythm with ECG and report abnormalities.
- Assess skin/nail bed color, capillary refill, and peripheral pulses, and report abnormalities.

- Give cardiovascular medications and oxygen as ordered.
- Reduce myocardial oxygen demand by utilizing comfort measures to reduce pain and anxiety and keeping the body at an appropriate temperature.
- Provide explanations for procedures, the condition, and its treatment.

Cancer

Cancer is identified by the tissues affected, the speed of cell growth, the appearance of the affected cells, and the location.

Cancer Classification

Tumor Type	Character	Origin
Fibroma	Benign	Connective tissue
Lipoma	Benign	Fat tissue
Carcinoma	Cancerous	Tissue of the skin, glands, and digestive, urinary, and respiratory tract linings
Sarcoma	Cancerous	Connective tissue, including bone and muscle
Leukemia	Cancerous	Blood, plasma cells, and bone marrow
Lymphoma	Cancerous	Lymph tissue
Melanoma	Cancerous	Skin cells

Seven Warning Signals of Cancer (American Cancer Society)

- Change in bowel or bladder habits.
- A sore that fails to heal.
- Unusual bleeding or discharge.
- Thickening or lump in breast or other tissue.
- Indigestion or swallowing difficulties.
- Obvious change in wart or mole.
- Nagging cough or hoarseness.

Cancer Prevention Methods

- Genetic testing.
- Healthy lifestyle.
- Protectant foods.
- Vaccines.

Diagnostic Tests

- Biopsy (surgical removal of tissue cells).
- Laboratory tests, such as blood, serum, and urine tests; bone marrow aspiration; and tumor markers.
- Cytological study (Pap smears).
- Radiological procedures, such as x-rays, contrast media x-ray studies, computed tomography (CT).
- Nuclear imaging procedures, such as the positron emission tomography (PET) scan.
- Ultrasound procedures.
- Magnetic resonance imaging (MRI).
- Endoscopic procedures.
- Tumor staging and grading.

Treatment

- Surgery.
- Radiation therapy.
- Chemotherapy.

Nursing Interventions

- Assess the meaning of quality of life to the client; assess suicide risk.
- Assess if client has any pain including onset, location, duration, and character; ask client to rate pain on a scale from 0 to 10 with 0 being the absence of pain and 10 being the worst pain.
- Administer analgesics as ordered; monitor pain relief every 2 to 4 hours.
- Monitor level of sedation and respiratory status if opioid dose is increased.

- Use nonpharmacological interventions once the pain is controlled with medication.
- Monitor lab tests daily, such as white blood cells, complete blood count, and platelets.
- Use good hand washing technique before interacting with the client.
- Teach client about not being around people who have colds or infections.
- Assess for signs of bleeding: bruising, petechiae, bleeding gums, tarry stools, and black emesis.
- Teach the client about gentle mouth care including no flossing, using a soft toothbrush, and wearing properly fitting dentures.
- Instruct the client not to take any salicylates or nonsteroidal anti-inflammatory medications to prevent bleeding.
- Instruct the client to use an electric razor.
- Monitor food and fluid intake and output every 8 hours.
- Give nutritional supplements as ordered by the physician.
- Give medications for nausea, vomiting, and diarrhea as ordered by the physician.
- Provide small, high-calorie meals to help reduce nausea.
- Administer pain medication before meals so the client can be comfortable while eating.

Cardiovascular Disorders

Angina Pectoris

- **Types:** Stable angina, variant angina, unstable angina, silent ischemia.
- **Causes:** Any event that increases oxygen demand can cause an angina attack, such as large meals, exercise, cold, stimulant drugs.
- **Signs/Symptoms:** Heaviness, tightness, squeezing, viselike, or crushing pain in the center of the chest; feelings of impending doom; pale, diaphoretic, or dyspneic.
- **Diagnostic Tests:** ECG, exercise electrocardiogram, graded exercise testing, stress echocardiography, chemical stress testing, radioisotope imaging, coronary angiography, biological markers.
- **Nursing Interventions:**
  - Assess the risk factors.
  - Obtain vital signs, oxygen saturation, and ECG to provide a baseline status.

- Notify physician of ECG changes.
- Consult the physician for pain management.
- Administer analgesics or aspirin, oxygen, and sublingual nitroglycerin.
- Remain with the client and reassess the pain in 5 minutes after the administration of medication.
- Promote rest and decrease anxiety for the client with chest pain.
- Teach client and family members the importance of weight reduction; a low-fat, low cholesterol diet; and stress reduction, which helps to slow the disease progression.
- Teach the client and family members the importance of taking medications used for angina: vasodilators, calcium channel blockers, and beta blockers.
- For clients with unstable angina, teach the client and family members the importance of taking the "Fab Four" of cardiac drugs (antiplatelets, statins, ACE inhibitors, and beta blockers) as ordered by the physician.

Arteriosclerosis

- **Causes:** Nonmodifiable factors: age, gender, ethnicity, genetics predisposed for hyperlipidemia; modifiable factors: diabetes mellitus, hypertension, smoking, obesity, sedentary lifestyle, increased serum homocysteine levels, increased serum iron levels, infection, depression, hyperlipidemia, excessive alcohol intake.
- **Signs/Symptoms:**
  - Vascular: capillary refill greater than 3 seconds, diminished peripheral pulses, dry skin, loss of hair on extremities, pallor in nail beds, thickened nails, leg cramps.
  - Cardiac: chest pain, diaphoresis, dizziness, fatigue, nausea, shortness of breath, weakness, arterial bruits.
- **Diagnostic Tests:** Cholesterol, triglycerides, arteriogram, blood glucose level.
- **Nursing Interventions:**
  - Encourage client to follow a low-fat diet. Provide information from the American Heart Association for guidelines and diets to decrease fat and cholesterol intake.
  - Teach about the risks of smoking and exposure to second-hand smoke. Provide information from the American Cancer Society for smoking cessation programs.

- Encourage client to increase activity as ordered by the physician.
- Teach the purpose of lipid-reducing medications, if the physician orders drug therapy.

Cardiac Dysrhythmias

- **Arrhythmia**: An irregularity or loss of rhythm of the heartbeat.
- **Dysrhythmia**: An abnormal, disordered, or disturbed rhythm. This is the most accurate term for abnormal rhythms.
- **Ventricular Dysrhythmias:** Include premature ventricular contractions, ventricular tachycardia, ventricular fibrillation, and asystole.
- Therapeutic interventions for cardiac dysrhythmias include cardiac pacemakers, defibrillation, automatic external defibrillators, implantable defibrillator, cardioversion, and ablation.
- **Nursing Interventions:**
  - Take apical and radial pulses every 2–4 hours.
  - Monitor blood pressure and urinary output.
  - Monitor mental status every 2–4 hours.
  - Listen to lung sounds every 2–4 hours.
  - Administer oxygen as ordered.
  - Encourage the client to get adequate rest and not to exceed activity tolerance.
  - Administer medications as ordered and monitor for side effects.
  - Explain the purpose of therapeutic interventions.

Cerebrovascular Accident

- **Causes:** Ischemia: embolism or thrombosis; hemorrhage: rupture of a cerebral blood vessel.
- **Signs/Symptoms:** Vary depending on the area of the brain affected; visual disturbances, language disturbances, weakness or paralysis on one side of the body, difficulty swallowing; included with hemorrhagic stroke, rapid deterioration, drowsiness, severe headache.
- **Diagnostic Tests:** Use of the Cincinnati Prehospital Stroke Scale (CPSS); CT scan; ECG; CBC; metabolic panel; blood typing; prothrombin time (PT) and international normalized ratio (INR); stool and emesis checks for blood; carotid Doppler testing; cerebral angiogram.

■ **Nursing Interventions:**
  ■ Assess neurological status, vital signs, lung sounds, cough, respirations, and skin frequently.
  ■ Administer anticoagulants and monitor coagulation studies if ordered.
  ■ Position client to maintain airway and suction if cough is ineffective.
  ■ Implement seizure precautions.
  ■ Support affected extremities with pillows, maintain good body alignment, reposition every 2 hours to prevent complications, and consult PT and OT for impaired mobility.
  ■ Keep client NPO until swallowing can be evaluated.
  ■ Assess for facial weakness, inability to completely close mouth, and drooling.
  ■ If swallowing appears to be intact, have client swallow a sip of water from a cup before offering other foods or fluids. Observe for coughing, choking, or noisy lung sounds.
  ■ Provide safety by implementing measures to prevent aspiration by staying with client, ensure that client is fully alert before feeding, have client in semi-Fowler's position or in a chair before eating, avoid the use of straws, use a thickening agent if swallowing study recommends, place food on unaffected side of mouth, instruct client to swallow twice after each bite, check the client's mouth for pocketing of food, and have suction equipment ready.
  ■ Notify physician if client is unable to take in adequate calories orally.
  ■ Assist with the insertion of a feeding tube if ordered.
  ■ Assess bowel and bladder continence, client's ability to perform ADLs, difficulties in verbal communication, and thought processes.
  ■ Implement skin care measures, provide assistance with toileting according to the client's usual schedule, encourage highest level of independence possible by facilitating client's ability to do ADLs, assist client with learning to use nondominant side of body, and implement measures to facilitate communication.
  ■ Explain what happened to the client. Explain tests, procedures, and care activities.
  ■ Discharge activities include referring to social worker for assistance with financial resources, rehab, and/or home health.

Coronary Artery Disease

- **Causes:** Primary cause of coronary artery disease is atherosclerosis.
- Acute coronary syndrome is used to describe the manifestations of coronary artery disease.
- **Signs/Symptoms:** ACS: unstable angina, non-ST elevation myocardial infarction, and ST elevation. Possible MI may occur.
- **Diagnostic Tests:** Cholesterol, triglycerides, arteriogram, blood glucose level.
- **Nursing Interventions:**
  - Prepare client for possible invasive procedures, such as percutaneous transluminal coronary angioplasty, coronary athrectomy, coronary artery stents, myocardial revascularization–coronary artery bypass graft, and transmyocardial laser revascularization.
  - Provide appropriate care after invasive procedures.

Hypertension

- **Types:**
  - Primary, or essential hypertension.
  - Secondary hypertension.
  - Isolated systolic hypertension.
- **Signs/Symptoms:** Elevated blood pressure; may complain of a headache, bloody nose, severe anxiety, or shortness of breath.
- **Diagnostic Tests:**
  - Prehypertensive state is greater than systolic of 120 and diastolic of 80.
  - Hypertension is the average blood pressure, for two or more readings on different dates, greater than systolic of 139 and diastolic of 89.
- **Complications:**
  - Heart failure.
  - Coronary artery disease.
  - Atherosclerosis.
  - Myocardial infarction.
  - Stroke.
  - Renal failure.
  - Eye damage.

Hypertensive emergency: SBP greater than 180 mmHg and DBP greater than 120, along with possible target-organ dysfunction,

Hypertensive urgency is severe elevation of BP without the target-organ dysfunction.

- **Nursing Interventions:**
  - Provide client and family information about disease processes, including risk factors, complications, and treatment regimen.
  - Help clients identify their risk factors and ways to change their lifestyles. Identify barriers that may prevent clients from making the necessary lifestyle changes.
  - Assist client by providing referral sources for financial assistance in obtaining medications and refills.
  - Teach client to take medications as prescribed and not to stop.
  - Instruct the client not to double up on medication if a dose was skipped.
  - Teach client to change positions slowly to prevent falls.

Myocardial Infarction

- **Causes:** Any event that increases oxygen demand can cause a myocardial infarction, such as large meals, exercise, cold, stimulant drugs.
- **Signs/Symptoms:** Crushing chest pain, shortness of breath, dizziness, nausea, sweating, fatigue, cramping in chest, anxiety, feeling of impending doom, falling.
  - Symptoms found in women: epigastric or abdominal pain, chest discomfort, pressure, burning, arm, shoulder, neck, jaw, or back pain, discomfort/pain between shoulder blades, shortness of breath, fatigue, indigestion or gas pain, nausea or vomiting, sleep disturbances.
- **Diagnostic Tests:** ECG, CBC, serum cardiac troponin I or T; serum myoglobin, serum CK-MB, serum magnesium and potassium, vital signs, oxygen saturation, intake and output.
- **Nursing Interventions:**
  - Inform the client and family members about the importance of seeking treatment within 5 minutes of unrelieved chest pain.
  - Inform the client and family members that the American Heart Association recommends chewing one uncoated adult aspirin at the onset of chest pain.

- Teach client and family members the importance of calling emergency medical services. Explain that the client should not drive to the hospital alone.
- Once in the hospital, monitor the location, duration, intensity, and radiation of pain.
- Monitor vital signs.
- Provide oxygen immediately, usually at 2 L/min via nasal cannula.
- Administer the Fab Four medications as ordered by the physician and observe client carefully for side effects.
- Inform the client that bed rest is required.
- Provide a bedside commode for bowel movements.
- Inform client and family members about the importance of cardiac rehabilitation.

Endocrine Disorders

Hyperparathyroidism

- **Causes:** Hyperplasia or a benign tumor of the parathyroid glands, or it may be hereditary; possibly cancer.
- **Signs/Symptoms:** Increased serum calcium levels, fatigue, depression, confusion, increased urination, anorexia, nausea, vomiting, kidney stones, and cardiac dysrhythmias, gastric secretion resulting in abdominal pain and peptic ulcer; bone and joint pain pathological fractures; coma and cardiac arrest could occur.
- **Diagnostic Tests:** Serum calcium levels, phosphate, and PTH levels; radiograph; nuclear scanning.
- **Nursing Interventions:**
  - Monitor for and report signs or symptoms of calcium imbalance promptly.
  - Encourage oral fluids and strengthening and weight-bearing exercises.
  - Provide a safe environment for ambulation; assist the client with ambulation if necessary.
  - Encourage smoking cessation.
  - Teach client and family members the importance of which symptoms to report and use of long-term medications.
  - Teach client and family members how to administer hydrocortisone intramuscularly in an emergency.

Hypoparathyroidism

- **Causes:** Hereditary; accidental removal of the parathyroid glands; hypomagnesemia.
- **Signs/Symptoms:** Hypocalcemia causes neuromuscular irritability; tetany; numbness and tingling of the fingers and perioral area, muscle spasms, and twitching; lethargic, calcifications may occur in the eyes and brain, leading to psychosis; cataracts; bone changes; convulsions; death.
- **Diagnostic Tests:** Chvostek's and Trousseau's signs; serum calcium levels, PTH levels, increased serum phosphate, radiograph.
- **Nursing Interventions:**
  - Monitor for signs of tetany and report immediately to the physician.
  - Make sure a tracheostomy set, endotracheal tube, and intravenous calcium.
  - Teach client and family members of the importance of eating a high calcium diet.
  - Teach the client about the importance of diet and medication therapy and follow-up laboratory testing.

Hyperthyroidism

- **Causes:** Graves' disease is thought to be caused by an autoimmune disorder; pituitary tumor; thyroid hormone; radiation exposure; heredity.
- **Signs/Symptoms:** Hypermetabolic state, such as heat intolerance, increased appetite with weight loss, increased frequency of bowel movements; nervousness, tremor, tachycardia, and palpitations; heart failure may occur; thickening of the skin on the anterior legs and bulging of the eyes; photophobia and blurred or double vision.
- **Diagnostic Tests:** Thyroid levels; TSH level; thyroid scan; palpitation of the thyroid; TSI (thyroid-stimulating immunoglobulin) is present.
- **Nursing Interventions:**
  - Monitor vital signs, especially the temperature.
  - Administer acetaminophen as ordered.
  - Apply cooling blanket, as ordered. Set to 1–2°F below current temperature, and wrap extremities with towels.

- Provide a low-fiber, low-sodium diet and small frequent meals of bland foods (bananas, rice, applesauce).
- Monitor electrolytes and for signs of dehydration.
- Keep skin clean and dry; apply skin barrier cream.
- Monitor weight weekly.
- Consult dietitian for high-calorie diet with six meals.
- Administer medications, such as sedatives, to help client rest, as ordered.
- Administer antianxiety medications, as ordered.
- Administer lubricating saline eye drops as ordered to keep the eyes from drying.
- Instruct client to use dark, tight-fitting glasses.
- Gently tape eyes shut with nonallergic tape for sleeping.
- Elevate the head of the bed.
- Teach client and family members about the importance of notifying the physician immediately if eye pain or vision changes occur.
- Teach client and family members about the importance of taking prescribed medications and the importance of routine follow-up laboratory testing.

Hypothyroidism

- **Causes:** Caused by congenital defect, inflammation of the thyroid gland, or iodine deficiency; autoimmune disorder, pituitary or hypothalamic lesion, postpartum pituitary necrosis.
- **Signs/Symptoms:** Reduced metabolic rate resulting in fatigue, weight gain, bradycardia, constipation, mental dullness, feeling cold, shortness of breath, decreased sweating, and dry skin or hair. Heart failure may occur; hyperlipidemia; decreased libido, erectile dysfunction.
- **Diagnostic Tests:** Thyroid hormone levels, TSH levels, serum cholesterol and triglycerides.
- **Nursing Interventions:**
  - Administer medications, as ordered.
  - Assist with self-care activities, allowing time for client to rest between activities.
  - Monitor and record bowel movements.
  - Increase fluid intake to eight 8-ounce glasses of water daily if cardiovascular status is stable.

- Teach client and family members the importance of adding fiber to diet, such as fresh fruit, vegetables, and bran.
- Teach client and family members the importance of observing the skin for breakdown, avoiding the use of soap on dry areas, and using nondrying lotion following bath.
- Consult the dietitian, as ordered, to develop a diet.

Type I Diabetes Mellitus

- **Causes:** Autoimmune response; genetic predisposition; virus.
- **Signs/Symptoms:** Polyuria; polydipsia; polyphagia; fatigue; blurred vision; headache; abdominal pain.
- **Diagnostic Tests:** Fasting plasma glucose, HbA1c (glycosylated hemoglobin), oral glucose tolerance test; additional testing for complications.

Type II Diabetes Mellitus

- **Causes:** Heredity; obesity; may have had a recent life stressor, such as the death of a family member, illness, or loss of a job.
- **Signs/Symptoms:** Same as Type I diabetes mellitus.
- **Diagnostic Tests:** Same as Type I diabetes mellitus.
- **Nursing Interventions for Type I and Type II Diabetes Mellitus:**
  - Assess client's and family members' understanding of knowledge of diabetic self-care.
  - Teach client and family members about appropriate glucose levels and what actions need to be taken if glucose levels are too high or too low.
  - Teach client and family members how to assess glucose levels before meals and at bedtime or as ordered by health care provider, the importance of having meals taken appropriately with medications, and the replacement of any uneaten foods to prevent hypoglycemia.
  - Teach client and family members the technique for administering insulin.
  - Teach client and family the causes, prevention, recognition, and treatment of hypoglycemia and hyperglycemia.
  - Assess client's and family members' ability to see and manipulate syringe, glucose monitor, and other equipment.
- Consult dietitian and social worker if ordered.

Acute Pancreatitis

- **Causes:** Associated with excessive alcohol consumption, biliary disease, gallstones, blunt trauma, thiazide diuretics, estrogen, opioids, corticosteroids, and excessive serum calcium.
- **Signs/Symptoms:** Dull abdominal pain, guarding, a rigid abdomen, hypotension or shock, respiratory distress, low-grade fever, dry mucous membranes, tachycardia, nausea, vomiting, and jaundice may occur.
- **Diagnostic Tests:** Serum amylase and lipase, urine amylase, complete chemistry panel, x-ray examination, CT scan, and ultrasonography.
- **Nursing Interventions:**
  - Monitor IV fluids, blood, or blood products, if ordered.
  - Administer antianxiety drugs, pain medication, and antiemetics as ordered.
  - If respiratory problems occur, administer oxygen as ordered.
  - Monitor nasogastric feeding, if ordered.
  - If client is NPO for a prolonged amount of time, the physician may order TPN.
  - Monitor intake and output.

Gallbladder Disorders

- **Causes:** Pooling of bile within the gallbladder; excessive cholesterol intake combined with a sedentary lifestyle; fasting; family history, obesity, diabetes mellitus, pregnancy, some hemolytic blood disorders, and bowel disorders.
- **Signs/Symptoms:** Elevated vital signs, vomiting, jaundice, epigastric pain, right upper quadrant (RUQ) tenderness, nausea, indigestion, positive Murphy's sign, pain begins suddenly after a fatty meal and lasts for 1–3 hours; heartburn, indigestion, and flatulence.
- **Diagnostic Tests:** WBC, serum amylase levels, abdominal x-ray exam, nuclear scan, sonograms.
- **Nursing Interventions:**
  - Assess the client for pain frequently.
  - Administer analgesics, antispasmodics or anticholinergics, and antiemetics as ordered.

- Provide comfort measures by positioning the client.
- Postoperatively monitor intake, output, daily weights, skin turgor, and T-tube drainage.
- Assess the client for the return of bowel sounds and passage of flatus.
- Monitor IV fluids and electrolytes as ordered while the client is on restricted oral intake.
- Assess for signs of jaundice, excessive itching, and excessive drainage or evidence of infection around the surgical incision.
- Encourage the client to cough and breathe deeply, and assist by splinting the abdomen.
- Teach client and family members the importance of staying on a high-protein, low-fat diet. After surgery, the client can slowly introduce fat back into the diet.

Hepatitis

- **Causes**: Caused by one of six viruses: hepatitis A virus (HAV); hepatitis B virus (HBV); hepatitis C virus (HCV); hepatitis D virus (HDV); hepatitis E virus (HEV); and hepatitis G virus (HGV).
- **Signs/Symptoms**: Three stages of loss of liver function:
  - **Prodromal stage**: Flulike symptoms of malaise, headache, anorexia, low-grade fever, dull RUQ pain, nausea, vomiting, diarrhea or constipation.
  - **Icteric stage**: Fatigue, anorexia, nausea, vomiting, malaise, jaundice, dark amber urine, clay-colored stools.
  - **Posticteric stage**: Client feels well during this time, but full recovery may take as long as 1 year.
- **Diagnostic Tests**: Elevated serum liver enzymes (ALT, AST), elevated serum bilirubin, HAV antigen; HBV antigen; HCV antigen; HDV antigen; abdominal x-ray exams; prothrombin time; erythrocyte sedimentation rate.
- **Nursing Interventions**:
  - Monitor weight and nutritional intake.
  - Provide a high-calorie, high-protein, high-carbohydrate, low-fat diet as ordered. Provide frequent, smaller meals.
  - Administer antiemetic drugs, antihistamines, and analgesics as ordered.

- Provide comfort measures by placing the client in an upright or sitting position to eat meals.
- Teach client and family members to avoid alcohol and vitamin supplementation unless specifically prescribed by the physician.
- Teach client not to scratch and to keep fingernails trimmed short.
- Provide comfort measures by keeping the room temperature at a comfortable level to decrease perspiration.
- Teach client and family members the necessity of proper home cleanliness, including hand washing after toileting and using soap and water to clean eating utensils, cookware, and food preparation surfaces.
- Teach client and family members the importance of adequate rest and proper nutrition, avoiding alcohol and other liver-toxic drugs.
- Teach client and family members how the disease spreads to others.

Liver Failure

- **Causes:** Excessive alcohol ingestion, massive exposure to hepatotoxins, viral hepatitis or infection; chronic inflammation and obstruction of the gallbladder and bile ducts; severe congestion of the liver from heart failure.
- **Signs/Symptoms:** Malaise, anorexia, indigestion, nausea, weight loss, diarrhea or constipation, dull aching RUQ pain, bruising of the skin, jaundice, severe pruritis, hepatorenal syndrome, blood clotting defects, ascites, portal hypertension, and hepatic encephalopathy.
- **Diagnostic Tests:** Liver serum enzymes, serum bilirubin, urobilinogen, serum ammonia, prothrombin time, abdominal x-rays, upper GI series, liver scan, esophagogastroduodenoscopy (EGD), liver biopsy.
- **Nursing Interventions:**
  - Weigh the client on admission and daily.
  - Monitor ascites by measuring and recording the client's abdominal girth.
  - Report any weight gain or increase in abdominal girth.
  - Monitor the client's vital signs every 4 hours; report any changes and any evidence of difficulty breathing or changes in mental status promptly.
  - Consult a dietitian as ordered.

- Provide client with a low-sodium diet and fluid restriction as ordered.
- Administer diuretics and analgesics as ordered.
- Assess the client's bowel sounds, abdominal distention, and evidence of bleeding at least once every 8 hours.
- Offer frequent mouth care.
- Administer vitamins or supplements as ordered.
- Assess level of consciousness and neuromuscular function frequently.
- Reorient the client to time and place frequently.
- Monitor client safety to prevent falls.
- Promote comfort by repositioning client every 2 hours.
- Monitor lab values and report abnormalities to physician.
- Monitor gastric secretions, stool, and urine at least every 8 hours, and report any signs of bleeding.
- Caution the client to use a soft-bristle toothbrush and an electric razor.
- Avoid suctioning the client if possible.
- Use a small-gauge needle for injections and apply direct pressure to all puncture sites.
- Teach client and family members the importance of avoiding hot, spicy, or irritating foods.
- Instruct the client to avoid forceful coughing or nose blowing, straining, vomiting, or gagging if at all possible.
- Teach client and family members the importance of avoiding narcotics, sedatives, and tranquilizers.

Gastrointestinal (GI) Disorders

Absorption Disorders

- **Causes:** Ileal dysfunction, jejunal diverticuli, parasitic disease, celiac disease, enzyme deficiency, bacterial infections, inflammatory bowel diseases.
- **Signs/Symptoms:** Weight loss; weakness; general malaise; frequent loose, bulky, foul stools that are gray in color; increased fat in the stool; abdominal cramping; excessive gas; and loose stools after eating milk products.

- **Diagnostic Tests:** CBC, upper GI series, D-Xylose absorption test, Sudain stain for fecal fat; 72-hour stool collection for fat.
- **Nursing Interventions:**
  - Assess normal pattern of defecation, diet, and fluid intake.
  - Administer medications as ordered.
  - Encourage client to drink 2 to 3 L of fluid per day.
  - Teach client and family members the importance of increasing fiber and bran in the diet and limiting caffeine.
  - Encourage the use of a food diary documenting foods and timing of symptom occurrence to help identify food triggers.

Appendicitis

- **Causes:** Obstruction resulting in an inflammatory response.
- **Signs/Symptoms:** Fever, increased WBCs, generalized pain in the upper abdomen. In later stages the pain is localized at the right lower quadrant midway between the umbilicus and the right iliac crest, along with nausea, vomiting, and anorexia.
- **Diagnostic Tests:** CBCs, ultrasound, CT scan.
- **Nursing Interventions:**
  - Instruct the client to remain NPO 12 hours prior to surgery.
  - Promote comfort until surgery by placing ice over the painful area and placing client in a semi-Fowler's position.
  - Prepare the client for being NPO after surgery until the GI begins to function.
  - Prepare the client for the possibility of having a nasogastric tube in place after surgery.
  - Monitor vital signs and assess the abdomen for signs of peritonitis.
  - Provide pain management and encourage early ambulation, coughing, deep breathing, and turning to prevent respiratory complications.

Diverticulosis and Diverticulitis

- **Causes:** Chronic constipation; decreased intake of dietary fiber.
- **Signs/Symptoms:** Generally asymptomatic. If symptoms occur, client exhibits signs of bowel changes, alternating between constipation

and diarrhea; steady or crampy pain in the left lower quadrant of the abdomen; bleeding may occur, along with weakness, fever, fatigue, and anemia; guarding and rebound tenderness.

- **Diagnostic Tests:** Sigmoidoscopy, colonoscopy, barium enema; if abscess is suspected, a CT scan is done.
- **Nursing Interventions:**
  - Educate the client and family members about the importance of increasing dietary fiber and preventing constipation.
  - If client is hospitalized, promote comfort measures by administering pain medication and antibiotics as ordered.
  - Once acute period is over, a progressive diet is ordered.
  - Monitor for signs of an intestinal perforation.
  - If surgery is required, prepare the client and family members for a possible temporary colostomy.
  - If the client does not have inflammation with the diverticulosis, instruct client and family members on the importance of adding fiber and bulk to the diet.
  - Instruct to increase fiber intake slowly to prevent excess gas and cramping.

Gastritis

- **Causes:** Alcohol, spicy foods, microorganisms, medications, stress, trauma, smoking, radiation, nasogastric suctioning, endoscopic procedures; chronic gastritis A is referred to as autoimmune gastritis; chronic gastritis B is associated with *Helicobacter pylori* bacterial infection.
- **Signs/Symptoms:** Abdominal pain, nausea, anorexia, abdominal tenderness, feeling of fullness, reflux, belching, hematemesis.
  - Chronic gastritis A: asymptomatic; may have difficulty absorbing vitamin B_{12}.
  - Chronic gastritis B: poor appetite, heartburn after eating, belching, sour taste in the mouth, nausea and vomiting.
- **Diagnostic Tests:** Type A and B are diagnosed by endoscopy, upper GI x-ray examination, and gastric aspirate analysis.
- **Nursing Interventions:**
  - Teach client and family members to identify causative factors that cause the gastritis.

- With the assistance of the dietitian, teach client and family members the importance of staying on a bland diet of liquids and soft foods as ordered by the physician.
- Teach client and family members the importance of taking medications ordered by the physician, including antibiotics for the *H. pylori* bacteria.

Gastroesophageal Reflux Disease (GERD)

- **Causes:** Conditions that affect the ability of the lower esophageal sphincter to close tightly.
- **Signs/Symptoms:** Heartburn, regurgitation, dysphagia, bleeding; possible aspiration.
- **Diagnostic Tests:** Barium swallow; endoscopy; pH monitoring of alkaline esophagus.
- **Nursing Interventions:**
  - Teach client and family members the importance of making lifestyle changes to help manage GERD, such as eating a low-fat, high-protein diet, and to refrain from caffeine, milk products, and spicy foods.
  - Teach client and family members the importance of taking medication even if symptoms are relieved.
  - Prepare client for surgical management, if ordered, by providing preoperative and postoperative instructions.

Intestinal Obstruction

- **Causes:** Two types: mechanical is caused by adhesions, twisting of the bowel, or strangulated hernia; paralytic is caused by abdominal surgeries, trauma, mesenteric ischemia, or infection.
- **Signs/Symptoms:**
  - Small-bowel obstruction: wavelike abdominal pain and vomiting. If obstruction is mechanical, high-pitched tinkling bowel sounds are heard proximal to the obstruction and are absent distal to it. If obstruction is nonmechanical, there is an absence of bowel sounds.
  - Large-bowel obstruction: develops slowly and depends on the location of the obstruction. Crampy lower abdominal pain, abdominal distention, vomiting, localized tender area, and mass may be palpated.

- **Diagnostic Tests:** Small-bowel obstruction: radiographic studies and CT scan; CBC; electrolyte panels; large-bowel obstruction: radiological examination.
- **Nursing Interventions:**
  - Prepare the client for surgery.
  - Give medications for pain as ordered.
  - Provide comfort measures by placing client in semi-Fowler's position and providing frequent mouth care.
  - Maintain NPO status until intestinal function resumes.
  - Monitor IV fluid replacement.
  - Provide postoperative care.
  - Instruct client to increase fluids if diarrhea occurs to prevent hydration.
  - If surgery is necessary to treat the intestinal colitis, prepare the client and family members for the postoperative experience.
  - Administer analgesics, antidiarrheals, and medications as ordered.
  - Document characteristics of stools, including color, consistency, amount, frequency, and odor.
  - Encourage bedrest.
  - Instruct client and family members about the importance of avoiding high-fiber foods, such as whole grains, raw fruits, vegetables, caffeine, alcohol, and nicotine.
  - Assess for signs of fluid deficit.
  - Provide comfort care by keeping perianal skin clean, dry, and protected with moisture barrier after each bowel movement.

Peptic Ulcer Disease

- **Causes:** *Helicobacter pylori* bacteria.
- **Signs/Symptoms:**
  - Gastric: intermittent high left epigastric or upper abdominal burning or gnawing pain, increased 1–2 hours after meals or with food. Variable pain pattern may be worse with food, antacids are ineffective. Client may be malnourished; hematemesis may occur.
  - Duodenal: intermittent midepigastric or upper abdominal burning or cramping pain, increased 2–4 hours after meals or in the middle of the night; relieved with food or antacids. Client is well nourished. Melena is more common than hematemesis. Anorexia, nausea/vomiting, bleeding.

■ **Diagnostic Tests:** Urea breath test; IgG antibody detection test; biopsy; culture, upper GI series; esophagogastroduodenoscopy.
■ **Nursing Interventions:**
  ■ Assess location, onset, intensity, characteristics of pain, nonverbal pain cues, and vital signs.
  ■ Administer antiulcer medications as ordered.
  ■ Provide small, frequent meals four to six times per day.
  ■ Encourage nonacidic fluids between meals.
  ■ Monitor for signs and symptoms of hemorrhage.
  ■ Monitor intravenous infusion as ordered.
  ■ Monitor lab values and report abnormalities to the physician.

Hematological and Lymphatic Disorders

Anemias

■ **Causes:** Dietary deficiencies; hemolysis; hereditary (thalassemia, sickle cell); aplastic anemia may be congenital or from exposure to toxics, chemotherapy medications, or use of cardiopulmonary bypass during surgery; bacterial and viral infections.
■ **Signs/Symptoms:** Pallor, tachycardia, tachypnea, irritability, fatigue, shortness of breath, peripheral neuropathy, inflamed tongue, spoon-shaped fingernails. Aplastic anemia: same as anemia; as disease progresses, tachycardia and heart failure may appear. Sickle cell: severe pain and swelling in the joints, abdominal pain, fever, renal failure.
■ **Diagnostic Tests:** CBC, serum iron, ferritin, and total iron-binding measurements; serum folate; bone marrow biopsy and analysis; blood smear that shows sickle-shaped RBCs; hemoglobin elec-trophoresis; erythrocyte sedimentation rate.
■ **Nursing Interventions:**
  ■ Monitor vital signs during exertion. If vital signs increase, reduce the activity level.
  ■ Assist the client with self-care activities, as needed, by placing articles within easy reach.
  ■ Encourage the client to limit visitors, telephone calls, and unneces-sary interruptions.

- Administer oxygen as ordered.
- Use safe practices when verifying client identification for blood transfusion.
- Monitor vital signs and adverse effects frequently during the blood transfusion.
- Teach the client and family members about the disease process and ways that foods can help correct nutritional deficiencies.
- Instruct the client and family members about the importance of taking the supplements as ordered.
- Teach the client and family members about the importance of lifelong injections of vitamin B_{12} if the client has pernicious anemia.
- Protect the client with pernicious anemia from injuries resulting from decreased sensation.
- If the client is taking iron supplements, teach the client and family members the importance of reporting adverse effects of iron supplements.
- If ordered, administer iron injections using the Z-track method.
- Administer liquid supplements with a drinking straw to avoid staining the teeth.
- Teach the client and family members the importance of preventing falls by changing positions slowly and assisting the client with ambulation.
- Teach the client and family members the importance of maintaining good oral hygiene; eating soft, bland foods; and using a soft tooth-brush for oral care.
- Monitor IV fluids for the client with sickle cell anemia.
- Apply warm compresses as ordered to the painful joints, cover the client with a blanket, and keep the room temperature higher than 72°F.
- Teach the client and family members to use warm compresses, avoid cold compresses, and avoid restrictive clothing.
- If the client with sickle cell anemia has severe pain, monitor for adverse effects of opioid analgesics.
- Administer acetaminophen for fever.
- Teach the client and family members to avoid using aspirin.
- Encourage the client to rest during the acute phase.

Disseminated Intravascular Coagulation (DIC)

- **Causes:** Can occur after major trauma; heatstroke; shock; snakebite; fat embolism.
- **Signs/Symptoms:** A catastrophic, overwhelming state of accelerated clotting throughout the peripheral blood vessels; all clotting factors become exhausted resulting in bleeding from nearly every bodily route.
- **Diagnostic Tests:** PT, PTT (prolonged), hemoglobin (decreased), BUN (increased); serum creatinine (increased).
- **Nursing Interventions:**
  - Early recognition and reporting of signs of bleeding are critical to survival.
  - Avoid trauma that may cause bleeding; do not dislodge clots from any site.
  - Provide a soft toothbrush and electric razor.
  - Avoid invasive procedures or intramuscular injections.
  - Avoid medications that interfere with platelet function (i.e., aspirin, NSAIDs).
  - Administer stool softeners to prevent straining during bowel movement.
  - Reposition client gently to avoid bruising.
  - Instruct client not to blow nose.

Hemophilia

- **Causes:** Hereditary, X-linked recessive lack of specific clotting factors. Hemophilia A is caused by a deficiency of Factor VIII (80% of cases). Hemophilia B is caused by a deficiency of Factor IX (15% of all cases).
- **Signs/Symptoms:** Females are carriers; males have the disorder; spontaneous bleeding; excessive bleeding in response to trauma; hemarthrosis.
- **Diagnostic Tests:** CBC, PT; PTT; genetic testing.
- **Nursing Interventions:** Same as DIC.

Hodgkin's Disease

- **Causes:** Cause unknown; possible viral, such as mononucleosis; possible genetic link; clients with AIDS or those taking immunosuppressive drugs are at high risk.
- **Signs/Symptoms:** Painless swollen lymph nodes; weight loss, generalized pruritis, cough, dysphagia, or stridor; fatigue, persistent low-grade fever, and night sweats; local to regional area of spread.
- **Diagnostic Tests:** Lymph node biopsy, bone marrow biopsy and aspiration, liver and spleen biopsies, chest x-ray, abdominal CT scan, lymphangiography, CBC, nodes staged based on Ann Arbor Clinical Staging Classification.
- **Nursing Interventions:**
  - Assess the amount of activity the client can tolerate. Assist with ADLs as necessary. Encourage client to rest between activities.
  - Provide oxygen therapy as ordered.
  - Assess client for signs and symptoms of infections and report immediately.
  - Teach client and family members the signs and symptoms of infection and when to report the symptoms to the physician.
  - Teach the client to avoid exposure to others with influenza, colds, or other infections.
  - Teach client and family members the importance of proper hand washing and good oral and personal hygiene.
  - If the client's spleen becomes enlarged, prepare the client for a possible splenectomy.
  - Provide postoperative care for the client who has undergone a surgical splenectomy.
  - Refer client and family members to a cancer survivor's support group.

Leukemia

- **Causes:** Malignant disease of the white blood cells.
- **Signs/Symptoms:** Fever; pallor; weakness; malaise; tachycardia; dyspnea; bone pain; headaches; confusion.
- **Diagnostic Tests:** CBC; bone marrow aspiration; lumbar puncture.

- Monitor vital signs every 4 hours.
- Monitor for signs of infection.
- Observe for signs of bleeding; same as DIC interventions.
- Assist in administration of chemotherapy, radiation, or bone marrow transplant.

Immune Disorders

Hypersensitivity Reactions

Type I Hypersensitivity Reactions

- **Causes:** Allergic reaction provoked by exposure to an allergen; secretion of active mediators such as histamine, leukotriene, and prostaglandin.
- **Signs/Symptoms:** Vasodilatation; increase in mucus production; allergic rhinitis; allergic asthma; atopic dermatitis (eczema); urticaria; anaphylaxis.
- **Diagnostic Tests:** Physical examination and history; skin testing.
- **Nursing Interventions:**
  - To identify the disorder early, monitor respiratory rate, depth, nasal flaring, or abdominal breathing.
  - Monitor the client for signs of restlessness, confusion, changes in the level of consciousness, changes in voice, or dysphagia.
  - Position the client in a high-Fowler's or semi-Fowler's position if respiratory problems occur.
  - Assess and document skin condition and whether lesions are present.
  - Teach client to keep fingernails short and clean to reduce the risk of infection from scratching.
  - Teach client to minimize scratching by applying clean, white cotton cloth over affected sites.
  - Teach client to rub gently over affected sites instead of scratching.
  - Teach client and family members about the importance of wearing a medical alert identification for allergies.
  - Encourage the client to avoid possible allergens to reduce reactions.

- If allergen is environmental, teach the client the importance of obtaining a prescription for an epinephrine pen and how to use it.
- For atopic dermatitis (eczema), teach the client the signs and symptoms of infection and the importance of using a humidifier during the winter months to prevent dryness, wearing cotton clothing to minimize irritation, and taking cool soaks to decrease pruritis.
- For urticaria, teach the client stress management and relaxation techniques.
- Teach client to follow the therapeutic regimen including prescribed medications and their correct usage.
- Document teaching and client understanding.

Type II Hypersensitivity Reactions

- **Causes:** Blood transfusion; incompatibility.
- **Signs/Symptoms:** Sudden onset of low back pain; chest pain; hypotension; fever; chills; tachycardia; wheezing; dyspnea; urticaria; anxiety; headache; nausea.
- **Diagnostic Tests:** Direct Coomb's test.
- **Nursing Interventions:**
  - **Prevention is crucial**.
  - Follow institutional policy about having two nurses check the blood once released from blood bank.
  - Double-check the client's name and identification bracelet in addition to checking the client's blood type in the chart, on the unit of blood, and on the paperwork with the unit of blood. This is usually done at the client's bedside.
  - Vital signs are taken before the beginning of the transfusion, every 15 minutes for the first hour, every 30 minutes for the second hour, then hourly until the transfusion is complete. Vital signs are taken at the completion of the transfusion.
  - If symptoms of a reaction occur, stop the blood transfusion immediately.
  - Keep the vein open with an infusion of normal saline.
  - Notify the physician and the blood bank immediately.
  - Remain with the client for support and continue monitoring symptoms and vital signs.
  - If a blood transfusion is incompatible, it is important to return the unused blood and tubing back to the blood bank for testing.

- If client develops respiratory problems, maintain airway and provide oxygen.
- Monitor vital signs and intake and output.
- Assess for pain and provide comfort measures.
- After a hemolytic transfusion reaction, tell the client and family members about the importance of informing future health care providers.

Type III Hypersensitivity Reactions

- **Causes:** Formation of antigen–antibody complexes, such as serum sickness seen after administering penicillin or sulfonamide.
- **Signs/Symptoms:** Severe urticaria; angioedema; fever; malaise; muscle soreness; arthralgia; splenomegaly; nausea, vomiting; diarrhea; lymphadenopathy.
- **Diagnostic Tests:** CBC; white cell count; sedimentation rate; complement assays.
- **Nursing Interventions:**
  - Administer antipyretics, analgesics, antihistamines, epinephrine, or corticosteroids as ordered to relieve symptoms.
  - Monitor pain using numeric scale.
  - Observe for signs of hypovolemia, restlessness, weakness, muscle cramps, headaches, or postural hypotension.
  - Monitor I&O to detect imbalances.
  - Encourage oral fluid replacement with hypotonic glucose-electrolyte solutions, such as sports drinks or ginger ale.
  - Administer IV fluids as ordered; monitor for fluid overload.

Type IV Hypersensitivity Reactions

- **Causes:** Transplant rejection; cell-mediated immune responses, such as contact dermatitis from poison ivy or poison oak or latex allergy.
- **Signs/Symptoms:** Reddened skin; pruritis; vesicular lesions; organ failure (if from transplant rejection).
- **Diagnostic Tests:** Physical examination and history; assessment of skin lesions; secondary infections.
- **Nursing Interventions:**
  - Contact dermatitis:
    - Implement same interventions as Type I hypersensitivity reactions.
    - Suggest tepid baking soda baths, colloidal oatmeal baths, and cool washcloths or cool baths to reduce itching.

- Transplant rejection:
  - Observe for signs of transplant rejection throughout the client's hospitalization.
  - Instruct the client and family members about the signs and symptoms of transplant rejection.
  - Instruct client and family members on the signs and symptoms of infection and when to notify the physician.
  - Instruct on the importance of staying on prescribed medication to prevent possible transplant rejection.
  - Instruct client and family members about the importance of avoiding people with colds or infections.

Autoimmune Disorders

Guillain-Barré Syndrome (GBS)
- **Causes:** Autoimmune response to a viral infection or vaccination.
- **Signs/Symptoms:** Divided into three stages: (1) ascending paralysis; (2) plateau; and (3) descending resolution: pain, cramping, numbness.
- **Diagnostic Tests:** History and physical; CSF, electromyography (EMG), nerve conduction velocity.
- **Nursing Interventions:**
  - Goal of nursing care is to support body systems until the client recovers.
  - Nursing care is the same as with other progressive neuromuscular disorders.

Multiple Sclerosis
- **Causes:** Autoimmune response; may be related to viral infections, heredity, and other unknown factors.
- **Signs/Symptoms:** Muscle weakness, tingling sensations, numbness, visual disturbances accompanied by pain, slurred speech, patchy blindness, vertigo, tinnitus, impaired hearing, nystagmus, ataxia, dysarrthria, dysphagia, constipation, spastic bladder, flaccid bladder, sexual dysfunction, anger, depression, euphoria.
- **Diagnostic Tests:** Based on history and physical exam; no specific test; cerebrospinal fluid (CSF) may be analyzed; MRI.

■ Teach client and family members the importance of avoiding risk factors (extreme heat and cold, fatigue, infection, physical and emotional stress, pregnancy) that can exacerbate symptoms and avoiding infection and illness by taking adequate rest periods, exercising, and eating a healthy diet.

Myasthenia Gravis

■ **Causes:** Chronic autoimmune process; may be initiated by a virus; disorders of thymus gland.
■ **Signs/Symptoms:** Progressive extreme muscle weakness especially during activity and improvement in muscle strength after rest; muscles are strongest in the morning.
■ **Diagnostic Tests:** History and physical exam; test using an intravenous injection of Tensilon; lab tests; EMG; pulmonary function tests.
■ **Nursing Interventions:**

■ Teach client and family members the importance of taking scheduled anticholinesterase drugs so that peak action occurs at times when increased muscle strength is needed for activities, such as meals and physical therapy.
■ Teach client and family members symptoms and treatment of myasthenic and cholinergic crises.
■ Teach client and family members the importance of adequate nutrition, methods to conserve energy, avoiding persons with infections and exposure to cold, and medications that need to be avoided.

Rheumatoid Arthritis (RA)

■ **Causes:** Cause unknown; however, there are indications that genetic predisposition and the environment play a role in triggering its development; an autoimmune response occurs.
■ **Signs/Symptoms:** Joint inflammation is bilateral and symmetrical; affected joints are slightly reddened, warm, swollen, stiff, and painful; morning stiffness lasting up to an hour; some may experience stiffness all day; activity decreases pain and stiffness; low-grade fever, malaise, depression, lymphadenopathy, weakness, fatigue, anorexia, and weight loss.
■ **Diagnostic Tests:** CBC; group of immunological tests (rheumatoid factor [RF]; red blood count [RBC]; C4 complement; erythrocyte

sedimentation rate [ESR], antinuclear antibody test [ANA]; C-reactive protein test [CRP]).

■ The higher the ESR, the more active the disease. X-ray exam, MRI, bone or joint scan, arthrocentesis.

■ **Nursing Interventions:**

    ■ Assess for pain, location, and severity of pain.

    ■ Administer analgesics and anti-inflammatory medications prior to activity.

    ■ Collaborate with interdisciplinary team, such as pain clinic, to explore alternative pain relief measures, such as surgery.

    ■ Assist with ADLs as necessary.

    ■ Encourage active ROM exercises; ensure proper positioning and joint alignment.

    ■ Teach client and family members the importance of using assistive devices.

    ■ Administer heat and cold therapy to aid in joint function.

Systemic Lupus Erythematosus (SLE)

■ **Causes:** Caused by the body rejecting "self"; cause unknown; may be a genetic link; infections, high stress levels, various hormones and drugs, and UV light have all been linked to triggering SLE; causes of death are kidney failure, heart failure, and central nervous system involvement.

■ **Signs/Symptoms:** No classic description; some only have skin and joints affected; others have devastating effects when the disease affects multiple body systems at the same time; classic feature is the characteristic raised, reddened butterfly rash found over the bridge of the nose; rash is usually dry and may itch; may be photosensitive, tends to worsen during an exacerbation; some clients have discoid (coinlike) skin lesions on other parts of the body; fever, arthralgia or arthritis, myalgia, malaise, weight loss, mucosal ulcers, and alopecia.

■ **Diagnostic Tests:** Skin lesions can be biopsied; ESR (erythrocyte sedimentation rate); ANA titers; SR protein (serine/arginine-rich proteins)

■ **Nursing Interventions:**

    ■ Teach client and family members the importance of preventing triggers to reduce exacerbations.

    ■ Teach client and family members the importance of minimizing exposure to the sun and wearing sunscreen, keeping immunizations up, and continuing with regular exercise.

- Teach client and family members the importance of taking medications, such as NSAIDs, acetaminophen, corticosteroids, antimalarials, and anticoagulants, and using topical creams and ointments as ordered.
- Teach client and family members the importance of avoiding people with infections if taking immunosuppressants.
- Teach client and family members the importance of proper hand-washing to prevent infections.

Immune Deficiencies

Primary Immunodeficiencies
- **Causes:** Genetic disorders.
- **Signs/Symptoms:** Recurrent infections; developmental delays; specific organ problems; autoimmune diseases.
- **Diagnostic Tests:** CBC with differential; immunoglobulin levels; T-cell function tests; B-cell function tests.
- **Treatments:** Depends on nature of abnormality; intravenous immunoglobulin; hematopoietic stem cell transplantation.

Acquired Immunodeficiencies
Human Immunodeficiency Virus (HIV)/Acquired Immunodeficiency Syndrome (AIDS)
- **Causes:** HIV.
- **Signs/Symptoms:**
  - *HIV:* Initially, no symptoms or acute retroviral syndrome; asymptomatic phase; immune system impairment: dyspnea, fever, weight loss, fatigue, night sweats, persistent diarrhea, oral or vaginal candidiasis ulcers, dry skin, skin lesions, peripheral neuropathy, shingles, seizures, or dementia.
  - *AIDS:* Diagnosed when CD4+ T-lymphocyte count is less than 200/μL or T-lymphocyte percentage is less than 14% of total lymphocytes or the presence of opportunistic infections and diseases.
- **Complications:** AIDS wasting syndrome; opportunistic infections; cancers; AIDS dementia complex.
- **Diagnostic Tests:** History and physical exam; HIV antibody tests; CB/lymphocyte count; CD4+/CD8+ T-lymphocyte count; viral load testing; viral culture.

Sexual Transmission

- CDC has recommended guidelines for counseling and testing people at risk for HIV.
- Women are at risk for developing HIV. Anal sex is the riskiest type of sexual act, for either gender, because it often results in tearing of the mucous membrane.
- Abstaining from sexual intercourse is the only sure way to prevent sexual exposure to HIV.
- A mutually monogamous sexual relationship is considered safe if both partners are not and will not be infected with HIV.

Parenteral Transmission

- Avoid injection drug use. Drug injection equipment must not be shared.
- Autologous (one's own) blood transfusion, when possible, is the safest type of transfusion to prevent HIV infection.

Perinatal Transmission

- Voluntary HIV pretest counseling and testing is offered during prenatal care for all pregnant women.
- Pregnant women who are HIV positive need to be encouraged to take antiretroviral therapy during pregnancy, labor, and delivery.
- Reduce infant's exposure to maternal blood by avoiding any procedure that increases the risk of exposure.
- At the time of delivery, pregnant women should be offered testing for HIV if they have not been tested or have not received prophylactic treatment.
- After delivery, the infant is given antiretroviral medication for 6 weeks.
- **Treatments:** Nonnucleoside reverse transcriptase inhibitors; nucleoside/nucleotide reverse transcriptase inhibitors; protease inhibitors; fusion inhibitors.
- **Nursing Interventions**
  - Assess client for sources of infections, risk factors, and presence of infections.
  - Caregivers should use standard precautions and strict aseptic technique for all clients and procedures.
  - If caregivers have respiratory infections, refrain from caring for client with AIDS.

- instruct visitors about techniques to avoid transmission of infections.
- Teach client and family members when to report signs of infections to health care provider.
- Perform frequent turning, optimum mobilization, protective mattress and chair pads, application of emollient to dry areas, and prompt treatment of any injuries to prevent skin injury.
- Teach strategies for skin care and avoidance of infection to client and family members.
- Encourage self-care as much as possible without tiring client.
- Encourage client to express feelings and concerns. Contact chaplain, counselor, or AIDS support worker at client request.
- Consult dietitian if diarrhea requires a dietary change.
- Mouth care is important. If painful lesions occur, the client should be encouraged to quit smoking (if smoker), use a soft toothbrush to promote comfort, and use viscous lidocaine to decrease pain during eating.
- Encourage the client to take medications exactly as instructed.
- Teach methods to prevent foodborne and waterborne infections.
- Financial resources may need to be addressed so that food and medications can be obtained.

Integumentary Disorders

Burns

- **Causes:** Open flames; hot objects; steam or scalding water; chemicals; electricity; radiation.
- **Signs/Symptoms:** Depends on depth of burn; severe pain; redness; singed hair; blisters; hoarse voice; coughing; restlessness; impaired thermal regulation; fluid and electrolyte imbalances; edema.
- **Diagnostic Tests:** Assessment of burn depth and total body surface area (TBSA) involved; CBC with differential; BUN; serum glucose; electrolytes; arterial blood gases; serum protein and albumin; urinalysis and urine culture; clotting studies; ECG; wound cultures.
- **Nursing Interventions:**
  - Check for depth of burn, percentage of total body surface area (TBSA) involved using "Rule of Nines"; and age of client.
  - Assess respiratory status; auscultate breath sounds every 15 minutes or as necessary.

- Monitor arterial blood gases and CO level; monitor for nasal flaring, retractions, wheezing, and stridor.
- Administer humidified 100% oxygen by tight-fitting mask for the breathing client.
- Elevate head of bed (if no cervical spine injuries or no history of multiple trauma).
- Provide appropriate pulmonary care: turn, cough, and deep breathe every 2–4 hours. Provide incentive spirometer every 2–4 hours, and suction frequently as needed.
- Obtain sputum cultures as ordered. Note amount, color, and consistency of pulmonary secretions.
- Administer bronchodilators and antibiotics as ordered.
- If heat is felt on wound, cool with tepid tap water or sterile water.
- Remove clothing and jewelry.
- Do not apply ice; cover client with clean sheet or blanket.
- Initiate immediate copious tepid water lavage for 20 minutes for all chemical burns, along with simultaneous removal of contaminated clothing. (Do not neutralize chemical because this takes too much time and resulting reaction may generate heat and cause further skin injury).
- Brush off dry chemicals before lavage.
- Use heavy rubber gloves or thick gauze for removal of clothing.
- Cleanse wound via bathing or showers.
- Do not wrap skin surface to skin surface; limit bulk of dressings; wrap extremities distal to proximal.
- Record intake and output hourly.
- Assess for signs and symptoms of hypovolemia (hypotension, tachycardia, tachypnea, extreme thirst, restlessness, disorientation).
- Monitor electrolytes, CBC.
- Administer IV fluids as ordered.
- Insert indwelling urinary catheters and monitor urine for amount, specific gravity, and hemochromogens.
- Administer osmotic diuretics as ordered; monitor response to therapy.
- Assess gastrointestinal function for absence of bowel sounds; maintain nasogastric tube.
- Assess level of pain; administer narcotics IV.

- Elevate burned extremities above the level of the heart; maintain comfortable environment.
- Assess pulses on burned extremities every 15 minutes. Use Doppler as necessary.
- Assess for numbness, tingling, and increased pain in burned extremity. Measure circumference of burned extremities.
- Apply burn dressing loosely.
- Assist with escharotomy as necessary.
- Use sterile technique with wound care.
- Maintain protective isolation with good hand-washing technique.
- Administer immunosuppressive medications as ordered: tetanus and gamma globulin.
- Perform wound care as prescribed, which may include the following: inspect and debride wounds daily; culture wound three times a week or at sign of infection; shave hair at least 1 inch around burn areas (excluding eyebrows); inspect invasive line sites for inflammation (especially if line is through a burn area).
- Continually assess for and report signs and symptoms of sepsis: temperature elevation; changes in sensorium; changes in vital signs and bowel sounds; decreased output; positive blood/wound cultures.
- Administer systemic antibiotics and topical agents as prescribed.

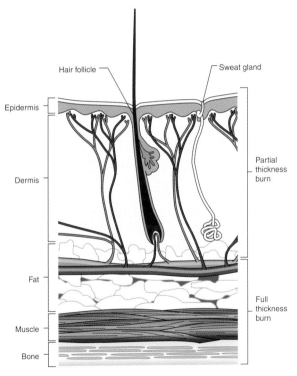

Partial- and Full-Thickness Burns

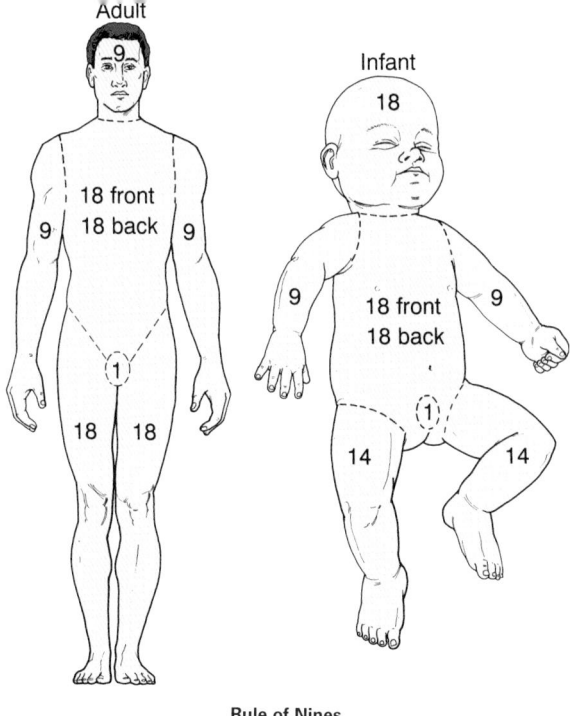

Rule of Nines

Inflammatory Skin Disorders

- **Causes:** From exposure to allergens or irritants, by heredity, or by emotional stress.
- **Signs/Symptoms:** Itching, rashes, and lesions may present as dry, flaky scales; yellow crusts; redness; fissures; macules; papules; and vesicles.
- **Diagnostic Tests:** History, symptoms, clinical findings, culture.
- **Nursing Interventions:**
  - Monitor skin condition regularly.
  - Cleanse the area as ordered by the physician, taking care not to further irritate the skin.
  - Provide cool moist compresses, dressings, or tepid tub baths.
  - Pat the skin dry rather than rub it.
  - Apply topical agents as ordered. Teach client how to apply topical agents.
  - Provide skin care at bedtime.
  - Encourage client to eat a high-protein diet, to use gloves or mitts especially at night, to keep fingernails short, to wear long sleeves or other appropriate covering, and to use a humidifier in the home.
  - Teach client and family members that application of slight pressure with a clean cloth may help relieve itching; inform of relaxation exercises.
  - Teach client and family members how to recognize changes, improvement, or flare-ups of the disorder; what symptoms to report to the health care provider; and measures to prevent future flare-ups if possible.

Skin Lesions

- **Causes:** Overexposure to ultraviolet rays, most commonly sunlight. Other factors include being fair skinned and blue eyed, genetic tendencies, history of x-ray therapy, exposure to certain chemical agents, burn scars, chronic osteomyelitis, and immunosuppressive therapy.
- **Signs/Symptoms:** Lesion is small pearly or translucent papule; lesion can appear as a single, crusted, scaled eroded papule; may be prone to oozing or bleeding.

■ **Diagnostic Tests:** Preliminary diagnosis is based on the appearance of the lesion; definitive diagnosis is made by biopsy.
■ **Nursing Interventions:**
  ■ Palpate lesions to determine texture, size, and firmness.
  ■ Document size, location, color, surface characteristics, pain; discomfort; itching; bleeding.
  ■ Provide same nursing care as care of cancer.
  ■ Prepare client for cryosurgery.

Musculoskeletal Disorders

Fractures

■ **Causes:** Trauma from either a fall or accident or some type of crushing injury; bone diseases can cause fractures.
■ **Signs/Symptoms:** May complain of tenderness over the site of the injury or more severe pain when moving the affected part of the body; the limb may be shortened because of contraction of the muscles pulling on the bone sections; range of motion is decreased; bruising may be present over a closed fracture; in an open fracture, one or more bone ends pierce the skin, causing a wound.
■ **Diagnostic Tests:** X-ray examination; CT scan; MRI; CBC; serum calcium levels.
■ **Nursing Interventions:**
  ■ Provide comfort measures for client during fracture management, which may include reduction or realignment of bone ends, immobilization of the fractured bone, prevention of deformity or further injury, preservation or restoration of function, promotion of early healing, and pain relief.
  ■ Monitor vital signs frequently.
  ■ Administer pain medication and anti-inflammatory medications as ordered.
  ■ Observe dressings, wounds, and pin sites for signs and symptoms of infection.
  ■ Monitor color of and measure wound drainage.
  ■ Teach client how to use a fracture bedpan.
  ■ Teach client how to transfer with bandages or a cast on extremity and ambulation techniques.

- Teach client how to use an overhead frame with a trapeze.
- Monitor client for and take measures to prevent complications of immobility by turning client every 2 hours; checking skin; keeping heels off the bed; teaching client to deep breathe and cough every 2 hours; and teaching the use of an incentive spirometer.
- Apply thigh-high elastic stockings or sequential compression device to unaffected limbs as ordered.
- Give anticoagulants as ordered.
- Ambulate client as early as possible as ordered.
- Remind client to practice leg exercises.
- Include other disciplines such as the physical therapist in promoting and teaching about ambulation as ordered.
- Assess for compartment syndrome if client is in a cast.

Muscular Dystrophy

- **Causes:** Genetic origin; exact cause is unknown.
- **Signs/Symptoms:** Difficulty walking, muscle weakness in arms, legs, and trunk; frequent falls, developmental delays, drooping eyelids, drooling, intellectual restriction, contractures, and skeletal deformities.
- **Diagnostic Tests:** Serum creatinine phosphokinase (CPK); electromyography (EMG); muscle biopsy, lactic dehydrogenase (LDH), isoenzymes, myoglobin (urine or serum), creatinine (urine or serum), CPK isoenzymes, aspartate aminotransferase (AST) levels; tests for gene mutation.
- **Nursing Interventions:**
  - Assess for muscle weakness, noting which areas are being affected and the severity of the weakness.
  - With the help of physical therapy, provide active and passive ROM exercises; provide assistive devices for mobility.
  - Teach client and family members the importance of the client doing as much as possible to help maintain muscle function.
  - Teach client and family members the importance of avoiding exposure to the cold and to persons with infections, and teach positions to help increase respiratory efficiency.

Osteoarthritis (Degenerative Joint Disease)

- **Causes:** Primary (idiopathic): cause unknown. Risk factors: aging, obesity, and physical activities. Secondary: results from trauma, sepsis, congenital anomalies, certain metabolic diseases, or systemic inflammatory connective tissue disorders.
- **Signs/Symptoms:** Joint pain and stiffness become severe, and client has problems with everyday activities; joint pain intensifies after physical activity but lessens following rest; client may complain of radiating pain and muscle spasms in the extremity innervated by the area affected.
- **Diagnostic Tests:** X-ray exams; CT scan, MRI, analysis of synovial fluid.
- **Nursing Interventions:**
  - Assess for pain, location, and severity of pain.
  - Administer analgesics and anti-inflammatory medications prior to activity.
  - Collaborate with interdisciplinary team, such as pain clinic, to explore alternative pain relief measures, such as surgery.
  - Assist with ADLs as necessary.
  - Encourage active ROM exercises; ensure proper positioning and joint alignment.
  - Teach client and family members the importance of using assistive devices.
  - Administer heat and cold therapy to aid in joint function and movement for those affected by RA.

Osteomyelitis

- **Causes:** Penetrating trauma; most common pathogens are *Pseudomonas aeruginosa, Staphylococcus aureus,* and *Proteus*; diabetes mellitus or peripheral vascular disease; hematogenous spread results from bacteremia, underlying disease, or nonpenetrating trauma; long-term intravenous catheters are primary sources of infection. Secondary: results from trauma, sepsis, congenital anomalies, certain metabolic diseases, or systemic inflammatory connective tissue disorders.

- **Signs/Symptoms:** Acute: fever, local signs of inflammation, such as tenderness, redness, heat, pain, and swelling over the area of infection. Chronic: ulceration, drainage, and localized pain
- **Diagnostic Tests:** Elevated WBC count, elevated erythrocyte sedimentation rate, positive bone biopsy for infection; blood culture, MRI; x-ray examinations, CT scans.
- **Nursing Interventions:**
  - If surgery is required, prepare the client for the removal of necrotic bone tissue.
  - If long-term antibiotic therapy is required, prepare the client for intravenous access.
  - Teach client and family members about the side effects, toxicity, interactions, and precautions for antibiotic therapy.
  - Teach client and family members of the importance of handwashing prior to dressing changes and how to avoid the spread of pathogens.

Osteoporosis

- **Causes:** Primary: not associated with another disease process. Secondary: is associated with a medical condition, such as hyperparathyroidism; having renal dialysis; drug therapy, such as steroids and certain antiseizure drugs, sleeping medications, hormones for endometriosis, or cancer drugs; prolonged immobility.
- **Signs/Symptoms:** Most women do not realize they have osteoporosis until they fracture a bone. May have a "dowager's hump" or kyphosis of the spine; client's height decreases and back pain may be present; may have difficulty finding clothes that fit comfortably.
- **Diagnostic Tests:** CT scan; bone density test; ultrasound; dual-energy x-ray absorptiometry (DEXA); serum calcium and vitamin D levels; serum phosphorus level; alkaline phosphatase level.
- **Nursing Interventions:**
  - Teach client and family members the importance of taking all prescribed medications used for prevention or treatment purposes, including calcium and vitamin D supplements, as ordered.
  - Teach client and family members foods that are high in calcium, such as dairy products and dark, green, leafy vegetables.
  - Teach client and family members to avoid excessive caffeine or alcohol.

- Teach client and family members the importance of performing weight-bearing exercises.
- Teach client and family members the importance of wearing well-supporting, nonskid shoes at all times and avoiding uneven surfaces that could contribute to falls.
- Teach client and family members the importance of creating a hazard-free environment, such as avoiding scatter rugs and slippery floors. Walking paths in the home must be kept free of clutter to prevent falls.

Neurological Disorders

Brief Neurological Assessment

Mental status	**Impression:** Observe affect, mood appearance, and grooming. **Speech:** Assess for clarity and coherence. **LOC:** Alert, lethargic, stuporous, or obtunded. **Orientation:** Person, place, and time.
Cranial nerves	*See Cranial Nerve Assessment.*
Motor	**Inspect:** Involuntary movements, muscle symmetry, atrophy. **Muscle tone:** Flex and extend wrists, ankles, and knees; slight, continuous resistance to passive movement is normal; note flaccid or rigid muscle tone.
Motor strength	Have client resist passive movement.
Reflexes	**Tendon Reflexes:** • 0 = Absent • 1+ = Diminished • 2+ = Normal • 3+ = Hyperactive without clonus • 4+ = Hyperactive with clonus **Babinski (Plantar Reflex):** Stroke the plantar surface of the sole of each foot with a reflex hammer; normal response is flexion of the toes; positive Babinski is extension of big toe and fanning of other toes. **Clonus:** Brisk dorsiflexion of foot with supported knee in partially flexed position; rhythmic oscillations = positive clonus.

Continued

Brief Neurological Assessment—cont'd

Gait/balance	Observe gait while client walks across room and returns. Have client walk heel-to-toe or on heels in a straight line. Have client hop in place on one foot.
Coordination	**Rapid Alternating Movements:** Instruct client to rapidly tap tip of thumb with tip of index finger. **Point-to-Point Movements:** Have the client touch his finger to his nose several times; alternate location of index finger. **Romberg Test:** Ask client to stand with feet together and eyes closed for 10 seconds. **BE PREPARED TO CATCH CLIENT**; test is positive if client becomes unstable.
Sensory	Ask client to close eyes; touch client with fingertip and/or toothpick to distinguish dull from sharp sensations; compare left and right sides of body.

Level of Consciousness

LOC	Characteristics
Alert	Awake; alert and oriented; understands written and spoken language; responds appropriately.
Confused	Disoriented to time, then place, then person; memory deficits; difficulty following commands; restless; agitated.
Lethargic	Oriented to time, place, and person; slow mental processes; sluggish speech; sleeps frequently but awakens when spoken to or touched; maintains wakefulness with sufficient stimulation.
Obtunded	Extreme drowsiness; responds with 1 or 2 words; follows very simple commands; requires vigorous stimulation to awake; stays awake for a few minutes at a time.
Stuporous	Minimal movement; responds unintelligibly; awakens briefly to repeated vigorous stimulation.
Coma	No response to verbal stimuli; does not speak.

Glasgow Coma Scale

Eyes open	Spontaneously: To command: 3 To pain: 2 Unresponsive: 1	Score
Verbal response	Oriented: 5 Confused: 4 Inappropriate: 3 Incomprehensible: 2 Unresponsive: 1	Score
Motor response	Obeys commands: 6 Vocalizes pain: 5 Withdraws from pain: 4 Abnormal flexion: 3 Abnormal extension: 2 Unresponsive: 1	Score
Total score:		

Cranial Nerve Assessment

Nerve		Name	Function	Test
I	S	Olfactory	Smell	Ask client to identify familiar odors.
II	S	Optic	Visual acuity/field	Assess visual acuity using Snellen chart; assess peripheral vision.
III	M	Oculomotor	Facial sensation/ muscles of mastication	Assess pupils for equality and reactivity to light.
IV	M	Trochlear	Pupillary reaction	Have client follow finger without moving head.
V	B	Trigeminal	Eye movement	Touch face with dull and sharp objects.

Continued

Cranial Nerve Assessment—cont'd			
Nerve		**Name**	**Function**	**Test**
VI	M	Abducens	Facial sensation/ muscles of mastication	Have client follow finger without moving head.
VII	B	Facial	Abduction of eye	Have client smile, wrinkle nose, puff cheeks, and differentiate between sweet and salty taste.
VIII	S	Acoustic	Hearing/ balance	Test hearing; have client stand with feet together, arms at side, eyes closed for 10 seconds.
IX	B	Glossopharyngeal	Swallowing; voice	Have client swallow and say "Ahh."
X	B	Vagus	Gag reflex	Elicit gag reflex.
XI	M	Spinal Accessory	Neck motion	Have client shrug shoulders or turn head against resistance.
XII	M	Hypoglossal	Tongue movement and strength	Have client stick out tongue and move it from side to side.

S, sensory only; M, motor only; B, both sensory and motor.

Amyotrophic Lateral Sclerosis (ALS or Lou Gehrig's disease)

- **Causes:** Unknown; may be genetic.
- **Signs/Symptoms:** Progressive muscle weakness, decreased coordination of arms, legs, and trunk; atrophy of muscles and twitching; muscle spasms may cause pain; difficulty with chewing and swallowing; inappropriate emotional outburst; speech becomes difficult; bladder and bowel function; pulmonary function becomes compromised as the condition worsens.
- **Diagnostic Tests:** History and physical exam; CSF analysis, EEG, nerve biopsy, EMG; blood enzymes.

- Reinforce information given by the physician to the client and family about ALS and its prognosis.
- Encourage family members to attend a support group.
- Teach client and family members the importance of rehabilitation using assistive devices and exercises to prevent complications, how to perform range of motion exercises, and need to avoid exposure to persons with infections.
- Provide end-of-life care.

Bell's Palsy

- **Causes:** Nerve trauma from a viral or bacterial infection; facial cranial nerve becomes inflamed and edematous.
- **Signs/Symptoms:** Seventh motor cranial nerve; loss of motor control, paralysis on one side of face; variable onset of symptoms; facial drooping and inability to close affected eye; drooling; loss of taste over anterior one-third of tongue; speech difficulties.
- **Diagnostic Tests:** History and physical exam; EMG.
- **Nursing Interventions:**
  - Assess level of pain.
  - Administer analgesics and eye drops or eye ointment as ordered.
  - Provide comfort measures by planning hygiene activities when pain relief is at its peak, teach client to chew on opposite side of face, and teach client to use electric razors instead of blades.
  - Provide warm, moist compresses prn; massage face; assist with facial exercises several times a day; and provide a facial sling.
  - Provide small, frequent meals; provide soft, easy-to-chew food at lukewarm temperatures; provide high-protein and high-calorie foods; avoid hot or cold drinks; and encourage oral hygiene after each meal and at bedtime.
  - Insert feeding tube on unaffected side if ordered.

Encephalitis

- **Causes:** Caused by viruses (e.g., West Nile virus); parasites, toxic substances, bacteria, vaccines, fungi, herpes simplex.
- **Signs/Symptoms:** Headache, fever, nausea, vomiting, general malaise, nuchal rigidity, confusion, decreased level of consciousness,

seizures, sensitivity to light, ataxia, abnormal sleep patterns, tremors, hemiparesis; cerebral edema.
- **Diagnostic Tests:** CT scan, MRI, lumbar puncture, electroencephalo-gram (EEG), cerebrospinal fluid analysis.
- **Nursing Interventions:**
  - Provide symptom control by administering anticonvulsants, antipyretics, corticosteroids, and analgesics as ordered.
  - Provide sleep aids or sedatives to reduce irritability.
  - Administer antiviral medications as ordered.

Headaches

- **Causes:**
  - *Tension or Muscle Contractions:* Associated with premenstrual syndrome, or psychosocial stressors, such as anxiety, emotional distress, or depression.
  - *Migraine:* Hereditary
  - *Cluster:* Vascular disturbance, stress, anxiety, and emotional distress; alcohol consumption may worsen the episodes.
- **Signs/Symptoms:**
  - *Tension or muscle contractions:* Radiation of pain to the crown of the head and base of the skull, with variations in location, is com-mon. Pressure, aching, steady, and tight.
  - *Migraine:* Throbbing, boring, viselike, and pounding; usually on one side of the head; triggers include specific foods, noise, bright light, alcohol, and stress.
  - *Cluster:* Headache begins suddenly, typically at the same time of night; tends to be unilateral, affecting the nose, eye, and forehead; bloodshot, teary appearance of the affected eye is common.
- **Diagnostic Tests:** History and symptoms; MRI; CT scan; skull x-ray, arteriogram; electroencephalogram; cranial nerve testing; lumbar puncture to test CSF.
- **Nursing Interventions:**
  - Assess for aggravating factors.
  - Teach client and family member the importance of identifying aggravating factors to reduce the frequency of attacks.
  - Encourage the client to use alleviating techniques such as biofeed-back or stress reduction.

- Provide a dark room and rest.
- Teach client and family members the importance of using relaxation techniques and warm, moist compresses.
- Teach client and family members the importance of medications, appropriate dosage, expected action, side effects, and consequences of misuse.

Meningitis

- **Causes:** Common organisms include *N. meningitides,* which causes meningococcal meningitis, and *S. pneumonia,* which causes pneumococcal meningitis.
- **Signs/Symptoms:** Headache, high fever, stiff neck, photophobia; petechiae on the skin and mucous membranes; nuchal rigidity, positive Kernig's and Brudzinski's signs; nausea and vomiting; encephalopathy, lethargy, and seizures.
- **Diagnostic Tests:** Lumbar puncture with CSF analysis, CBC, and C&S of nose and throat.
- **Nursing Interventions:**
  - Administer antibiotics, antipyretics, antiemetics, anti-inflammatory agents, and analgesics as ordered.
  - Avoid cooling the client to prevent shivering.
  - Provide a quiet environment for the client.
  - Place client in an isolation room to prevent the disease from spreading.
  - Teach client and family members the importance of preventing the client from hurting himself or herself.

Seizures/Epilepsy

- **Causes:**
  - *Acquired epilepsy:* Caused by traumatic brain injury and anoxic events.
  - *Idiopathic epilepsy:* Unknown cause.
- **Signs/Symptoms:** Symptoms correlate with the area of the brain where the seizure begins. Some experience an aura, which may be visual distortion, a noxious odor, or an unusual sound.
- **Diagnostic Tests:** EEG; sleep deprivation and flashing light stimulation.

■ **Nursing Interventions:**

■ Assess client for type of seizure and whether an aura is present.

■ Teach client and family members the importance of recognizing the aura and to get to safety if it occurs.

■ Teach client and family members the importance of moving away from furniture or other objects if an aura is present.

■ Teach client and family members the importance of wearing medical alert jewelry.

■ Help client and family members to identify conditions that trigger seizures, such as hypoglycemia, hypoxia, and hyponatremia.

■ Teach client and family members the importance of a consistent schedule of eating and sleeping.

■ Teach client and family members the importance of taking pre-scribed medication, dosage, side effects, and schedule and the importance of not stopping treatment suddenly.

■ Teach the client and family members the importance of regular blood tests if required.

■ If hospitalized, protect the client by padding side rails with commercial pads or bath blankets folded over and pinned in place.

■ Keep call light within reach.

■ Assist client when ambulating.

■ Keep suction and oral airway at bedside.

■ During a seizure, stay with client; do not restrain the client; protect from injury; loosen tight clothing; turn to side when able to prevent occlusion of airway or aspiration; suction if needed; monitor vital signs when able; be prepared to assist with breathing if necessary; and observe and document progression of symptoms.

Spinal Cord Injuries

■ **Causes:** Causes are similar to traumatic brain injury; diving into shallow water.

■ **Signs/Symptoms:** Flaccid paralysis and paresthesias (depending on level of the lesion); loss of reflex activity below the level of the lesion; spinal shock initially; risk for autonomic dysreflexia (injuries above sixth thoracic vertebra).

■ **Diagnostic Tests:** Plain radiographs; CT scan; MRI.

Nursing interventions:

- Monitor cough and lung sounds. Monitor for signs of autonomic dysreflexia: sudden high blood pressure, bradycardia, headache, pale skin below the injury, gooseflesh.
- If autonomic dysreflexia is present, immediately take the client's blood pressure and continue to monitor it every 5 minutes. Notify the physician.
- Teach client and family members the importance of identifying autonomic dysreflexia and ways to treat it.
- Suction client if unable to cough effectively.
- Place client in high-Fowler's position. Remove elastic stockings or any other garment that could prevent blood from pooling in the periphery.
- Catherize client if ordered.
- Check for impaction by performing a rectal examination.
- Include a suppository on a scheduled daily or every-other-day basis as ordered.
- Provide a high-fiber diet with adequate fluid intake as ordered.
- Implement bowel and bladder training program.
- Assess client's ability to move independently, feel pain, and feel pressure.
- Teach client and family members the importance of repositioning at least every 2 hours, the use of a pressure-reducing mattress, and preventive measures to reduce formation of pressure ulcers.
- If client is in traction or a halo brace, assess pin sites frequently. Keep sites clean and dry and report any sign of infection.
- Help client and family to identify resources. Consult a social worker to help client gain access to appropriate physical and financial assistance.

Respiratory Tract Disorders

Asthma

- **Causes:** Inherited tendency; triggered by allergens, such as pollen, foods, medications, animal dander, air pollution, molds, or dust mites; environmental irritants, smoking, respiratory or sinus infection; emotional upset, exercise; GERD.

- **Signs/Symptoms:** Chest tightness, dyspnea, difficulty in moving air in and out of the lungs; cough.
- **Diagnostic Tests:** Report of symptoms; physical examination; spirometry; allergy skin testing; serum IgE; eosinophil levels; arterial blood gases; PaO_2 decreases and $PaCO_2$ increases.
- **Nursing Interventions:**
  - Teach client and family members the importance of monitoring peak expiratory flow rate (PEFR) at home.
  - Help client identify triggers; teach client to avoid triggers, if possible.
  - If triggers cannot be avoided, instruct client and family members about the importance of using bronchodilators or mast cell inhibitor inhalers as prescribed.
  - Teach client and family members the importance of taking the inhaled corticosteroids to prevent symptoms.
  - Teach client and family members the importance of contacting the health care provider if the client uses more than two adrenergic MDI canisters per month.

Chronic Obstructive Pulmonary Disease (COPD)

- **Causes:** COPD is a group of pulmonary disorders; emphysema, chronic bronchitis, and asthma are part of COPD. Risk factors include smoking, exposure to secondhand smoke or industrial chemicals, and air pollution.
- **Signs/Symptoms:** Cough; chronic sputum production; dyspnea that occurs every day; worse with exercise; activity intolerance; crackles, wheezes, diminished breath sounds; barrel chest; use of accessory muscles; in late stages, clients may lose weight and become malnourished.
- **Diagnostic Tests:** Chest x-ray; CT scan; arterial blood gas analysis; CBC; sputum analysis; spirometry.
- **Nursing Interventions:**
  - Assess lung sounds, respiratory rate and effort, and use of accessory muscles.
  - Elevate head of bed or help client to lean on overbed table.
  - Administer oxygen at no more than 2 L/min unless ordered otherwise.

- Place a fan in the client's room.
- Teach client diaphragmatic and pursed-lip breathing.
- Teach client and family members the importance of not smoking.
- Encourage oral fluids to help decrease the thickness of the sputum.
- Use cool steam room humidifier.
- Administer expectorants as ordered.
- If client is unable to cough up secretions, suction per institution policy.
- Allow client to rest between activities. Bedrest may be necessary during acute dyspnea.
- Obtain bedside commode to help the client conserve energy.
- Assess if client has a living will or durable power of attorney for healthcare.

Influenza

- **Causes:** Various strains of flu viruses.
- **Signs/Symptoms:** Abrupt onset of fever, chills, myalgia, sore throat, cough, general malaise, and headache. It can last for 2–5 days, with malaise lasting up to several weeks.
- **Diagnostic Tests:** Viral cultures may be done, but results may take 5–10 days. Cultures may be done to rule out bacterial infection.
- **Nursing Interventions:**
  - Teach client and family members the importance of having yearly immunization to prevent the flu.
  - Teach client and family members that it takes 2 weeks for antibodies to build up after immunization.
  - Teach client and family members the importance of good hand-washing after contact with others, covering nose and mouth when coughing or sneezing, and not sharing eating or drinking utensils.

Pneumonia

- **Causes:** Bacterial, viral, fungal, aspiration, ventilator-associated pneumonia; hypostatic pneumonia; chemical pneumonia.
- **Signs/Symptoms:** Fever; shaking chills; chest pain; dyspnea; productive cough; purulent sputum; fatigue; sore throat; dry cough; nausea; vomiting.

- **Diagnostic Tests:** Chest x-ray; sputum and blood cultures; bronchoscopy.
- **Nursing Interventions:**
  - Teach client and family members the importance of obtaining the pneumonia vaccine every 5 years for prevention.
  - Administer broad-spectrum antibiotics after culture has been obtained as ordered.
  - Teach client and family members the importance of rest and fluids if the pneumonia is caused by a virus.
  - Teach client and family members the importance of taking prescribed expectorants, bronchodilators, and analgesics for comfort measures.
  - Teach client and family members the importance of taking prescribed nebulizer mist treatments or metered-dose inhalers.

Pneumothorax

- **Causes:** If it occurs without an associated injury, it is called a spontaneous pneumothorax. Underlying lung disease can cause secondary pneumothorax and hemothorax pneumothorax. Traumatic pneumothorax results from a penetrating chest injury. Other types are open pneumothorax, closed pneumothorax, and tension pneumothorax.
- **Signs/Symptoms:** Sudden dyspnea, chest pain, tachypnea, restlessness, anxiety; hypoxia, hypotension; trachea may deviate to the unaffected side; bradycardia; shock.
- **Diagnostic Tests:** History, physical examination, chest x-ray, arterial blood gases, oxygen saturation.
- **Nursing Interventions:**
  - Monitor client's breath sounds, vital signs, respiratory rate and depth, presence of dyspnea, chest pain, restlessness, or anxiety.
  - Report to physician any irregularities.
  - Provide comfort measures and pain management if client has a chest tube inserted and a water seal drainage system.

Pulmonary Embolism (PE)

- **Causes:** Risk factors of deep vein thrombosis (DVT) include surgical procedures done under general anesthesia, heart failure, fractures of lower extremities, immobility, obesity, oral contraceptive use, smoking, and history of DVT or PE; less common causes include fat emboli from compound fractures; amniotic fluid embolism during labor and delivery; air embolism from entry of air into the bloodstream.

- **Signs/Symptoms:** Sudden onset of dyspnea for no apparent reason; gasping for air; anxiety; tachycardia, tachypnea, and coughing; pleural friction rub; hemoptysis, pleuritic chest pain.
- **Diagnostic Tests:** Spiral CT scan; lung scan; pulmonary angiogram; chest x-ray exam; ECG; arterial blood gases; MRI; D-dimer.
- **Nursing Interventions:**
  - Monitor coagulation studies and report results to the physician.
  - Care is same for client taking anticoagulants.
  - Provide oxygen as ordered.
  - Teach client and family members the importance of maintaining anti-coagulant therapy for 3–6 months after being diagnosed with PE.
  - Teach client and family members the importance of obtaining regular PT and international normalized ratio (INR) to monitor Coumadin.
  - Prepare the client for an embolectomy, if ordered.

Sinusitis

- **Causes:** Most common infecting organisms are *Streptococcus* pneumonia and *Haemophilus* influenza; swelling caused by allergies, fungal infection, or intubation.
- **Signs/Symptoms:** Pain over the region of the infected sinuses; purulent nasal discharge; may experience pain over the cheek and upper teeth; may experience pain between and behind the eyes; may experience pain in the forehead; fever with or without generalized fatigue; foul breath.
- **Diagnostic Tests:** Uncomplicated sinusitis may be diagnosed by symptoms alone; x-ray exam, CT scan, MRI; culture and sensitivity of nasal discharge.
- **Nursing Interventions:**
  - Instruct the client to increase water intake to 8–10 glasses of water per day.
  - Explain to the client that the pressure may be relieved if sitting in a semi-Fowler's position.
  - Instruct client to use hot moist packs, analgesics, and prescribed medication as ordered.
  - Instruct client about the importance of taking all the prescribed medication and report to the physician if the pain becomes severe.

Tonsillitis/Adenoiditis

- **Causes:** Streptococcal, staphylococcal, *Haemophilus* influenza, and pneumococcal infection.
- **Signs/Symptoms:** Usually begins with a sore throat; headache, malaise, myalgia; nasal obstruction and nasal tone to voice if adenoids are infected.
- **Diagnostic Tests:** Throat culture; WBC, chest x-ray.
- **Nursing Interventions:**
  - Prepare the client for a tonsillectomy/adenoidectomy if the tonsillitis/adenoiditis is chronic or if breathing or swallowing is affected.
  - Provide postoperative care by keeping client in semi-Fowler's position, monitor for bleeding and airway obstruction, and provide comfort measures.
  - Avoid giving red-colored drinks. Encourage intake of cold fluids.
  - Keep suction equipment available for emergencies.

Sensory Disorders

Eye Disorders

Glaucoma

- **Causes:** Primary open-angle glaucoma (POAG) and acute angle-closure glaucoma (AACG) occur in people who have an anatomically narrowed angle; secondary glaucoma caused by infections, tumors, or injuries; congenital glaucoma is from developmental abnormalities.
- **Signs/Symptoms:**
  - AACG has a unilateral rapid onset; severe pain over affected eye, blurred vision, and rainbows around lights, eye redness, a steamy-appearing cornea, photophobias, tearing, nausea and vomiting with increased intraocular pressure.
  - POAG develops bilaterally. Onset is gradual and painless; later stages include mild aching in the eyes, headache, halos around lights, or frequent visual changes that are not corrected with eyeglasses.
- **Diagnostic Tests:** Tonometry, optic nerve is examined with ophthalmoscope, visual field examination, and infrared laser technology.

■ **Nursing Interventions:**
- Give analgesics as needed for acute glaucoma.
- Prepare client for possible eye surgery.
- Assist with self-care as needed.
- Teach client and family members the importance of not rearranging furniture without client knowledge; the importance of having regular eye examinations through dilated pupils; how to administer medications; the importance of using large, multicolored dot stickers placed on medication bottle with a corresponding direction card with a matching colored dot; and the importance of regular eye examinations for family members, who are at increased risk of developing glaucoma.

Infections and Inflammations of the Eye

- **Causes:** Caused by bacteria or viral; eye may be aggravated by allergens, chemical substances, or mechanical irritation.
- **Signs/Symptoms:** Visual disturbances, pain, redness, secretions, itchiness, sensation of pressure in eyes.
- **Diagnostic Tests:** Visual acuity, ophthalmoscopic examination of internal and external eye, Amsler grid, slit-lamp examination, tonometry.
- **Nursing Interventions:**
  - Assess for pain and any type of visual impairments.
  - Provide comfort measures by administering eye medications as ordered, administering antibiotics as ordered, applying warm or cool packs as ordered, and patching the affected eye.
  - Teach client and family members that when client has one eye patched, the perceptual field is altered so the client should not drive an automobile; discourage reading and watching television and encourage resting the eye by keeping the eye closed and listening to music or listening to an audio book.
  - Teach client and family members the importance of using caution when ambulating and reaching for things; teach not to wear contact lenses when the eye or surrounding structure is inflamed; and teach the importance of sterilizing contact lenses to prevent reinfecting the eye.
  - Teach client and family members the importance of prevention, care of the affected eye, medication administration, how to prevent spread of infection, and good eye hygiene.

Cataracts

- **Causes:** Contributing factors include age, ultraviolet radiation exposure, diabetes, smoking, steroid use, nutritional deficiencies, alcohol consumption, intraocular infections, trauma, and congenital defects.
- **Signs/Symptoms:** Painless, halos around lights, difficulty reading fine print or seeing in bright light, increased sensitivity to glare such as driving at night, double or hazy vision, and decreased color vision.
- **Diagnostic Tests:** Eye examination, visual acuity is tested for near and far vision; direct ophthalmoscope and slit-lamp microscope.
- **Nursing Interventions:**
  - Only treatment is surgical removal of the cloudy lens.
  - Prepare the client for eye surgery.
  - Teach client and family members that the depth perception may be affected by eye surgery, which can result in falls; ambulate with assistance and use clearly marked stairs. At home, beverages can be poured and stored in the refrigerator in single-serving glasses.
  - Teach client preoperative and postoperative activity restrictions, use of dark glasses to decrease the discomfort of photophobia, use of correct technique for administration of eye medications, reporting for medical follow-up as instructed, and protecting the eye from further injury.
  - In some types of cataract surgery, clients may be advised to avoid activities that might increase intraocular pressure, such as vomiting, coughing, sneezing, straining, or bending over or driving a car.
  - Teach client and family members the importance of seeking medical treatment if they experience sudden, worsening pain, increase in watery or bloody discharge, or sudden loss of vision.

Macular Degeneration

- **Causes:** Age-related; older than age 60 years; those with a family history; persons with diabetes; people who smoke; those frequently exposed to ultraviolet light, and Caucasians.
- **Signs/Symptoms:** Dry type: slow, progressive loss of central and near vision; each eye may be affected in different degrees; wet type: same loss of central and near vision, but the onset is sudden; loss can occur in one or both eyes; visual loss is described as blurred vision, distortion of straight lines, and a dark or empty spot in the central area of vision; may be a decreased ability to distinguish colors.

■ **Diagnostic Tests:** Visual acuity for near and far vision and an examination of the internal eye structures with ophthalmoscope; Amsler grid; intravenous fluorescein angiography.
■ **Nursing Interventions:**
  ■ If necessary, assist the client with assistive devices, such as handheld magnifying glasses, tableside magnifiers, television magnifiers, large-print items, phone dial covers with large numbers, talking watches, alarm clocks, and calculators.
  ■ Talk directly to client, not through a family member.
  ■ Explain any activity going on in the room or within client's auditory range.
  ■ Teach client and family members how to walk with the client and how to help him or her sit in a chair.
  ■ Refer client and family members to organization whose mission is to enhance the independence of persons with visual impairment.

Retinal Detachment

■ **Causes:** Can be precipitated by moderate trauma; can also occur in clients with sickle cell disease or diabetes mellitus; can occur in conditions, such as advanced hypertension, preeclampsia, or eclampsia, and from intraocular tumors.
■ **Signs/Symptoms:** Sudden change in vision; "flashing lights" are reported, then "floaters" are seen. Eventually, darkness occurs; loss of peripheral vision and loss of acuity in affected eye.
■ **Diagnostic Tests:** Indirect ophthalmoscope; slit-lamp examination
■ **Nursing Interventions:**
  ■ Prepare the client for the following methods of therapeutic interventions: laser reattachment, cryosurgery, electrodiathermy, sclera buckling, or pneumatic retinoplexy.

Ear Disorders

External Ear Disorders

■ **Causes:** Exposure to moisture, contamination, or local trauma; caused by bacterial or fungal pathogens.
■ **Signs/Symptoms:** Pain, pruritis, swelling, redness, drainage, lacerations, contusion, hematomas, abrasion, erythema, blistering, hearing loss, foreign body.

- **Diagnostic Tests:** CBC, audiometric, Rhinne's, Weber's, and whisper voice tests indicate conductive hearing loss with impacted cerumen and trauma; imaging studies to indicate extent of trauma.
- **Nursing Interventions:**
  - Assess for verbal and nonverbal signs of pain.
  - Administer analgesics as ordered.
  - Promote comfort by applying heat to the area, and offer liquid or soft foods.
  - Teach client and family members how to administer topical antibiotics and anti-inflammatory medications using aseptic technique; if a wick is inserted into the ear canal, monitor for drainage and report excessive drainage to health-care provider. Teach client how to care for ear and importance of keeping external ear clean and dry.

Hearing Loss

- **Causes:**
  - *Conductive hearing loss:* Cerumen, foreign bodies, infection, perforation of the tympanic membrane, trauma, fluid in the middle ear, cysts, tumor, and otosclerosis.
  - *Sensorineural hearing loss:* Complications of infections, ototoxic drugs, trauma, noise, neuromas, arteriosclerosis, and the aging process.
  - *Psychogenic hearing loss:* Precipitated by emotional stress.
- **Signs/Symptoms:** Difficulty understanding words or certain sounds, total deafness, changes in social and work activities, complains of people talking softly, speaks in a quiet or loud voice, answers questions inappropriately, avoids group activities, loss of sense of humor, appears aloof, complains of ringing or buzzing or roaring noise in ears.
- **Diagnostic Tests:** Abnormal Rhinne's and Weber's test results, audiometric testing indicates hearing loss.
- **Nursing Interventions:**
  - Assess hearing by inspecting ear canals for mechanical obstruction.
  - Enhance hearing by giving auditory cues in quiet environment.
  - Structure environment to compensate for hearing loss.
  - Introduce assistive devices such as hearing amplifiers, telephone amplifiers, telephones with extra-loud bells, written communication, and sign language.
  - Refer to specialized clinicians and hearing loss organizations.

Inner Ear Disorders

- **Causes:** Viral or bacterial pathogens.
- **Signs/Symptoms:** Vertigo, tinnitus, and sensoneural hearing loss, nystagmus, pain, fever, ataxia, nausea, vomiting, and beginning nerve deafness.
- **Diagnostic Tests:** CBC, Rinne's, Weber's.
- **Nursing Interventions:**
  - Instruct the client to avoid turning the head quickly to help alleviate the vertigo.
  - Institute fall precautions to help prevent injury.
  - Promote safety by ensuring that the client's environment is safe and free of obstacles. Environmental hazards, such as throw rugs, electrical cords in walkways, and poor lighting, should be removed by the family.
  - Assess for signs of headache or fullness in the ears.
  - Teach client and family members on correct dosage and administration of medications; to avoid using alcohol, caffeine, and tobacco; to call for assistance when ambulating; and to remain on bedrest until symptoms are relieved.

Middle Ear Disorders

- **Causes:** Inflammation of nasopharynx causes otitis media.
- **Signs/Symptoms:** Fever, earache, and feeling of fullness in affected ear following upper respiratory infection; nausea, vomiting, mastoid tenderness; otoscopic exam reveals reddened, bulging tympanic membrane; progressive hearing loss; vertigo; disorientation.
- **Diagnostic Tests:** CBC, ear cultures, audiometric, Rhinne's, Weber's, and whisper voice tests.
- **Nursing Interventions:**
  - Teach client and family members the importance of preventing spread of infection; the importance of never inserting anything into ear canal; how to correctly remove cerumen; take all prescribed antibiotics even if symptoms are relieved; ways to equalize ear pressure by yawning or performing jaw-thrust maneuver; avoid trauma to the ear, loud noise exposure, and environmental or occupational conditions.
  - Ensure that client knows how to administer ear drops and ear ointment.

- Teach client and family members the importance of seeking further medical attention if the client's pain worsens, hearing decreases, or drainage from ear is present.
- If surgery is indicated, prepare client with preoperative and postoperative instructions as needed.

Surgery

Preoperative Phase

Nursing Interventions

- Instruct the client not to take food or fluids past midnight the night before surgery.
- Inform clients that they may brush their teeth or rinse their mouth if no water is swallowed.
- If client is scheduled for an abdominal or intestinal surgery, prepare the client for an enema.
- Prepare client for the postoperative phase while the client is alert and ready to learn.
- Teach client about postoperative exercises to decrease complications, such as coughing and deep breathing, using incentive spirometry, doing leg exercises, turning and repositioning; also instruct client how to safely get out of bed.
- Inform client and family members about procedures and surgical routines.
- Allow clients to express any concerns.
- Inform the physician if clients express extreme anxiety or fear.
- Check to make sure that the informed consent has been signed.
- The informed consent involves three elements: (1) The physician must inform the client in understandable terms about the diagnosis, the treatment, the outcome, and any risks or complications that may occur. It is not within the nurse's scope of practice to provide this information. (2) The consent must be signed before analgesics or sedatives are given. (3) Consent must be signed voluntarily.
- Prepare the client for surgery.
- Send the client's chart, inhaler medications for those with asthma, and glasses or hearing aids to the surgical holding area.
- After client has left for the surgical holding area, prepare the client's room and equipment.

- Chest x-ray.
- Oxygen saturation.

Serum Tests

- Arterial blood gases.
- Bleeding time.
- Blood urea nitrogen.
- Creatinine.
- Complete blood cell count.
- Electrolytes.
- Fasting blood glucose.
- Pregnancy.
- Partial thromboplastin time.
- INR, prothrombin time.
- Type and cross match.

Urine Tests

- Pregnancy.
- Urinalysis.

Intraoperative Phase

Nursing Interventions

- Attention is given to the client's safety and special needs. For example, if a client is tall, a longer operating table may be needed.
- A surgical cart is prepared for the client ahead of time.
- Items, such as needles and sponges, are counted before surgery and after the incision has been closed to ensure that items have not been left inside the client.
- Electrical equipment is checked for proper functioning.
- Client allergies are rechecked.
- If hair needs to be removed, hair should be removed with electric clippers. Then the skin should be prepped with a solution that the client is not allergic to.
- Prep the skin using a circular motion from inside to outer edge.

Postoperative Phase

Nursing Interventions

- Admission assessment is done when the client is transferred from the surgical suite to the postanesthesia care unit (PAC).
- Priority areas for assessment are respiratory status and patency of airway; vital signs including SaO_2; level of consciousness and responsiveness; surgical site incision/dressing/drainage tubes; and pain level and pain management.
- If client had general anesthesia, maintain oxygen therapy as ordered.
- Encourage deep breathing.
- Give analgesics carefully and monitor for respiratory depression.
- Ensure that the client maintains a patent airway.
- Use jaw-thrust method to manually open client's airway.
- If client begins gagging, turn client on his or her side, unless it is contraindicated.
- Have suction equipment available.
- Check dressings and incisions for color and amount of drainage.
- Maintain IV fluids as ordered.
- Monitor intake and output.
- Maintain extremities in proper alignment and keep side rails up.
- Once client has been transferred to the unit, keep encouraging deep breathing and coughing every hour while the client is awake during the first postoperative day.
- Place incentive spirometer within client's reach, and encourage hourly use while awake.
- Turn client at least every 2 hours.
- Have client ambulate as soon as possible as ordered.
- Provide medications for comfort measures, such as analgesics and antiemetics.
- Maintain sterile technique for dressing change.
- Notify physician immediately if the bandage has bright-red drainage, remains sanguineous after a few hours, or is profuse.
- Encourage leg exercises hourly while the client is awake.
- Apply knee-high or thigh-length antiembolism stockings as ordered.
- Avoid pressure under the knee from pillows, rolled blankets, or prolonged bending of the knee and elevate legs.

- Measure and record client's output. Assess if the client is voiding small, frequent amounts.
- Notify physician if client is uncomfortable, has a distended bladder, or has not voided within the specified time frame postoperatively.

Urinary Disorders

Glomerulonephritis

- **Causes:** Immunological abnormalities, toxins, vascular disorders, and systemic diseases.
- **Signs/Symptoms:** Fluid overload with oliguria, hypertension; electrolyte imbalances edema; periorbital edema; flank pain.
- **Diagnostic Tests:** Urinalysis, dark urine or cola-colored, foamy urine from protein, creatinine; urea level elevated.
- **Nursing Interventions:**
  - Teach client and family members the importance of following the physician's order of sodium and fluid restrictions.
  - Teach client and family members the importance of taking pre-scribed diuretics, antihypertensives, and antibiotics as ordered.
  - If necessary, prepare the client for dialysis.

Renal Calculi

- **Causes:** Family history of stones, chronic dehydration, infection, dietary factors, immobility.
- **Signs/Symptoms:** Costovertebral angle pain, groin pain, renal colic, flank pain radiating to genitalia, hematuria, anuria, restlessness, pallor, temperature, diminished or absent bowel sounds with ileus.
- **Diagnostic Tests:** Urinalysis, crystals and urine pH, 24-hour renal creatinine clearance, BUN, creatinine, KUB reveals most calculi, retrograde pyelography, and ultrasound.
- **Nursing Interventions:**
  - Assess the client's pain and administer pain medication as ordered.
  - Prepare the client for surgical intervention, if ordered.
  - Monitor patency of drains and catheters in preoperative and post-operative clients.

- Encourage fluid intake unless contraindicated.
- Provide comfort measures by applying heat to flank area.
- Monitor vital signs to identify the postoperative complications of bleeding.
- Strain urine through gauze or strainer.
- Monitor urine output, color, clarity, and odor.
- Assess for signs of infection, such as an elevation in temperature, chills, or cloudy and foul-smelling urine.
- Teach client and family members the importance of identifying the relationship between activity and stones.
- Teach client and family members the importance of maintaining a fluid balance of 3,000 mL per day.
- Teach client and family members about medications used to prevent recurrence of renal stones.

Renal Failure (RF)

- **Causes:** Acute RF: hypotension, vascular obstruction, glomerular disease, acute tubular necrosis. Chronic RF: decreased urine output, acute renal failure symptoms appear rapidly, fatigue, nausea and vomiting, shortness of breath, platelet dysfunction.
- **Signs/Symptoms:** Fluid overload with oliguria, hypertension; electrolyte imbalances edema; periorbital edema; flank pain.
- **Diagnostic Tests:** Urinalysis, elevated BUN, creatinine, urine Na levels less than 10 mEq/L; acidosis, anemia, electrolyte abnormalities, elevated K, Mg levels, hypertension, pericarditis, platelet dysfunction, dialysis.
- **Nursing Interventions:**
  - Monitor intake and output, vital signs, signs for edema, serum protein and albumin levels, and signs of fluid overload.
  - Teach client and family member the importance of weighing daily.
  - If the weight gain is more than 2 pounds, then notify the physician.
  - Teach client and family members the importance of maintaining sodium and fluid restrictions as ordered.
  - Teach client and family members the importance of observing the skin for open areas and signs of infection.

- Teach client and family members the importance of bathing with tepid water, oils, or oatmeal and applying lotion to skin after bathing.
- Teach client and family members the importance of watching for signs of bleeding, how to prevent injury to self, how to practice good handwashing techniques, and when to report to the physician.
- Administer antiemetics before meals, erythropoietin, and antibiotics, if ordered.
- Prepare client for surgical intervention, such as obtaining a vascular access, and for dialysis.

Urinary Tract Infections (UTIs)

- **Causes:** *Escherichia coli*; obstruction, sexual intercourse; urinary catherization; reflux of urine; previous UTIs; aging.
- **Signs/Symptoms:** Urinary urgency, frequency, dysuria, flank pain, fever, chills, costovertebral tenderness, cloudy urine with casts, bacteria, WBCs, urine is positive for nitrites.
- **Diagnostic Tests:** Urinalysis culture greater than 100,000 bacteria, elevated WBCs, elevated sedimentation rate, increased neutrophils.
- **Nursing Interventions:**
  - Administer antibiotics and antispasmodic agents as ordered.
  - Administer estrogen cream to elderly clients to prevent future UTIs.
  - Instruct client and family members about the importance of taking all prescribed medications, forcing fluids, and returning for a follow-up urinalysis or culture after the antibiotic course is complete to ensure that the infection is gone.
  - Encourage voiding every 3 hours.
  - Teach client and family members the importance of avoiding cola, coffee, tea, and alcohol.
  - Teach client and family members the importance of drinking cranberry juice or taking vitamin C 500 mg to 1000 mg per day.
  - Instruct client to apply heating pad to suprapubic area to relieve discomfort.
  - Instruct client to empty bladder as soon as the urge is felt and after sexual intercourse.

- Teach client and family members the importance of avoiding bubble bath and scented toilet paper, which can be irritating.
- Instruct client to practice good perineal hygiene and to wipe front to back.
- Teach client and family members the importance of wearing cotton underwear.
- Teach client and family members the signs and symptoms of UTIs and when to report these symptoms to the physician.

Obstetrics

Prenatal/Antepartum Period: Fertilization to Start of Labor

Signs of Pregnancy		
Presumptive	**Probable**	**Positive**
Amenorrhea	Positive pregnancy test	Fetal heart beat
Breast tenderness	Uterine enlargement	auscultated
Quickening	Hegar's sign (softening of lower	Fetal movement
Nausea/vomiting	uterine segment)	palpated per
Urinary frequency	Goodell's sign (softening of cervix)	practitioner
	Chadwick's sign (bluish hue to	Ultrasound
	cervix/vagina)	confirmation
	Braxton Hicks contractions	

Pregnancy Testing

- **Urine Pregnancy Test:** Detects human chorionic gonadotropin (hCG).
- **Serum Pregnancy Test:** Useful in monitoring expected increase of hCG; detects hCG as early as 9 days postconception.
- **Ultrasound:** Confirms presence of gestational sac, fetal pole, and fetal cardiac activity; validates location of pregnancy (intrauterine vs. ectopic).

Predicting the Date (Nagele's Rule)	
Calculation:	**Example:**
Add **7 days** to the first day of the last normal menstrual period (LNMP).	1st day of LNMP: 10/14/01
Add **9 months**.	Add 7 days = 10/21/01
	Add 9 months = 7/21/02

Pregnancy Facts

- Pregnancy lasts approximately 40 weeks or 280 days.
- Amniotic fluid averages about 1,000 mL at term.
- Dilatation is the widening of the cervical os and canal.
- Effacement is the shortening and thinning of the cervix.
- Stages of fetal development include embryo (most critical; weeks 3–8) and fetus (from week 9 until delivery).
- Supine hypotension: caused by compression of vena cava; relieved by lying in a lateral recumbent position.
- Uterus: becomes abdominal organ by week 16.

Trimesters of Pregnancy

- **1st trimester**: From conception to 12 weeks' gestation.
- **2nd trimester**: From 13 to 27 weeks' gestation.
- **3rd trimester**: From 28 to 40 weeks' gestation.

Fundal Height Guidelines	
Gestation	**Fundal Height**
12 weeks	Just above symphysis pubis
16 weeks	Halfway between symphysis pubis and the umbilicus
20 weeks	At the umbilicus
21–36 weeks	Fundal height generally matches weeks of gestation in centimeters

Warning Signs During Pregnancy

- **Vaginal bleeding**: Abortion; placenta previa; abruptio placentae; preterm labor.
- **Leakage of vaginal fluid**: Premature rupture of amniotic fluid; incontinence of urine.
- **Dysuria**: Urinary tract infection.
- **Headache/altered vision**: Pregnancy-induced hypertension (PIH).
- **Abdominal cramping**: Preterm labor.
- **Severe epigastric pain**: PIH.
- **Decreased fetal movement**: Fetal demise.
- **Elevated temperature**: Infection.
- **Persistent vomiting**: Hyperemesis gravidarum.

Medication Pregnancy Risk Categories (FDA)

Category A	Adequate; no known increased risk of fetal abnormalities.
Category B	No adverse effects in animal studies/no human studies or adverse effects in animal studies/none in human studies.
Category C	Adverse effects in animal studies/no human studies or no animal or human studies.
Category D	Human studies show adverse fetal effects; maternal benefit may outweigh fetal risk in serious or life-threatening situations.
Category X	**Contraindicated**; human and/or animal studies show evidence of serious fetal abnormalities; fetal risks far outweigh maternal benefit.

Comparison of True and False Labor

True Labor	False Labor
Cervix dilates	Cervix unchanged
Contractions increase in intensity and frequency	Contractions irregular and decrease with change of position/activity
Leaking amniotic fluid; bloody show	No evidence of change in vaginal discharge
Low back pain; menstrual-like cramps	Mostly abdominal and groin discomfort

Intranatal Period: During Labor and Birth

Stages of Labor
- **Stage I:** From onset of contractions through full effacement and dilatation of cervix; lasts 8 to 18 hours.
  - *Latent phase:* 0–3 cm dilated.
  - *Active phase:* 4–7 cm dilated.
  - *Transition phase:* 8–10 cm dilated.
- **Stage II:** From full dilatation of cervix until delivery of baby; lasts 15 to 90 minutes.

- **Stage III:** From birth of baby until expulsion of placenta; lasts up to 20 minutes.
- **Stage IV:** First 1 to 2 hours after expulsion of placenta.

Electronic Fetal Monitoring	
Baseline	**Heart Rate Between Contractions**
Normal	120–160 bpm (can be higher for periods of less than 10 min).
Tachycardia	Sustained FHR greater than 160 bpm for 10 min. Common etiologies can include early fetal hypoxia, immaturity, amnionitis, maternal fever, and terbutaline (Brethaire®).
Bradycardia	Sustained FHR less than 120 bpm for 10 min. Common etiologies can include late or profound fetal hypoxia, maternal hypotension, prolonged umbilical cord compression, and anesthetics.

Short-Term Fetal Heart Rate Variability (One of the Most Important Indicators of Fetal Well-Being)	
Absent	0–2 variations per minute (abnormal); ominous sign; indicates hypoxia and/or acidosis; requires immediate delivery.
Minimal	3–5 variations per minute (abnormal); may indicate fetal sleep, stress, or effect of narcotic or anesthetic agents.
Moderate	6–25 variations per minute (normal).
Marked	More than 25 variations per minute (abnormal); may suggest acute hypoxia; maternal ephedrine administration, or uterine hyperstimulation.

Decelerations (Decrease in Fetal Heart Rate)

Timing	Etiology	Management
Early: starts and stops with contraction.	Head compression	Observation
Late: starts after contraction begins and ends after contraction ends.	Uteroplacental insufficiency	Lateral position; stopping or slowing Pitocin; oxygen, IV fluids; C-section if not corrected
Variable: occurs at unpredictable times during contractions	Cord compression	Lateral or Trendelenburg position; oxygen; C-section if not corrected

Intranatal Period: Complications

Abruptio Placentae

- **Causes:** Premature separation of placenta from uterus.
- **Signs/Symptoms:** Painful vaginal bleeding; rigid abdomen; shock; nonreassuring fetal signs.
- **Nursing Interventions:**
  - Assess signs and symptoms: bleeding, pain, uterine activity.
  - Obtain vital signs (VS) and fetal heart rate (FHR).
  - Monitor intake and output (I&O).
  - Obtain serum studies for disseminated intravascular coagulation (DIC): PT and PTT as ordered.
  - Maintain bed rest; administer oxygen and IV fluids; and assist RN in administration of blood products.
  - Prepare for cesarean birth.

Breech Presentation

- **Causes:** Multiple fetuses; abnormal volume of amniotic fluid; fetal anomalies; uterine abnormalities; previous cesarean section.
- **Types:**
  - *Frank breech:* Buttocks come first (65%–75% of breech presentations).
  - *Complete breech:* Baby sitting cross-legged with feet beside buttocks.

188

- *Footling breech:* One or both feet come first (common with premature fetuses).
- *Kneeling breech:* Baby in kneeling position (extremely rare).

■ **Signs/Symptoms:** Fetal heart tone above umbilicus; meconium without nonreassuring fetal signs.

■ **Nursing Interventions:**
  - Assess signs and symptoms, vital signs, nonreassuring fetal signs, and progress of labor.
  - Provide pain relief for "back labor."
  - Set up for both vaginal and cesarean birth.
  - Provide emotional support.
  - Administer nitroglycerin for rapid uterine relaxation if head becomes trapped.

Dystocia (Difficult Childbirth)

■ **Causes:** Uncoordinated uterine activity; abnormal fetal lie or presentation; cephalopelvic disproportion.

■ **Signs/Symptoms:**
  - *Maternal S&S:* exhaustion; extreme pain; increased pulse; contractions with increased frequency and decreased intensity; weakness; inefficient or stopped contractions; cervical trauma.
  - *Fetal S&S:* increased HR; nonreassuring signs; head molding; caput succedaneum; cephalohematoma; fetal demise.

■ **Nursing Interventions:**
  - Assess S&S, progress of labor, maternal VS, infection, and status of fetus.
  - Monitor response to oxytocin, if prescribed.
  - Administer pain relief measures.
  - Assist with x-ray and ultrasonography to identify pelvic size.
  - Have oxygen and resuscitation equipment nearby.

Meconium-Stained Amniotic Fluid

■ **Causes:** Post-term delivery; fetal distress.

■ **Signs/Symptoms:** Visualization of meconium in the amniotic fluid.

■ **Nursing Interventions:**
  - Suction nose and mouth with bulb syringe prior to delivery of the shoulders to prevent meconium aspiration.
  - Observe infant for signs of hypoxia or respiratory distress.
  - Have oxygen and resuscitation equipment nearby.

Placenta Previa

- **Causes:** Unknown; placenta attaches to the uterine wall close to or covering the cervix; usually occurs in the 3rd trimester.
- **Signs/Symptoms:** Painless, bright-red bleeding; soft uterus; anemia.
- **Nursing Interventions:**
  - Maintain bed rest; perform no vaginal examinations.
  - Monitor VS, FHR, and blood loss.
  - Obtain ultrasound confirmation.
  - Administer IV and transfusions for excessive blood loss as prescribed.
  - Administer betamethasone to increase fetal lung maturity; prepare for preterm birth or cesarean birth.

Premature Rupture of Membranes (PROM)

- **Causes:** Bacterial infection; defect in structure of amniotic sac, uterus, or cervix.
- **Signs/Symptoms:** Fluid leaking from vagina; amniotic fluid confirmed with fern and nitrazine tests.
- **Nursing Interventions:**
  - Establish time of rupture.
  - Avoid unnecessary vaginal examinations.
  - Assess for cord compression, FHR, maternal VS, and S&S of infection.
  - If at term and no labor within 12–24 hours, labor is induced.
  - If less than 37 weeks of gestation, maintain bed rest, administer prophylactic antibiotics, and assist with amnioinfusion of isotonic saline to decrease risk of cord compression.

Preterm Labor

- **Causes:** Cervical incompetence or inflammation; uterine abnormalities; infection; uteroplacental insufficiency.
- **Signs/Symptoms:** Contractions between 20th and 37th week, with 2-cm dilatation and 80% effacement; contractions every 10 min lasting 30 sec or longer.
- **Nursing Interventions:**
  - Maintain lateral recumbent position and quiet environment; administer tocolytic agents to suppress labor.
  - Administer betamethasone (Celestone®) to decrease severity of respiratory distress syndrome 24–48 hours before if birth appears probable.

- Assess FHR, maternal VS, and progress of labor; decrease BP with tocolytics.
- Treat respiratory depression with $MgSO_4$.
- Treat tachycardia with terbutaline and ritodrine.

Prolapsed Cord

- **Causes:** Usually concurrent with rupture of amniotic sac.
- **Signs/Symptoms:** Prolonged variable decelerations and baseline bradycardia; observation of cord protruding through cervix.
- **Nursing Interventions:**
  - Gently lift presenting part away from cord, which relieves pressure.
  - Provide oxygen.
  - Elevate client's hips while on side to increase placental perfusion.
  - Discourage pushing.
  - Assess FHR.
  - Notify physician immediately.
  - Prepare for possible cesarean birth.

Postpartum Period: After Birth

General Information

- Monitor for signs of postpartum hemorrhage and shock.
- If client is preeclamptic, assess blood pressure every hour.
- Client may have a slight fever (100.4°F) for the first 24 hours. Temperature greater than 101.4°F indicates an infection.
- Urinary retention is likely to occur postpartum; encourage fluids and monitor I&O for the first 12 hours.
- Encourage early ambulation; instruct client to change position slowly because postural hypotension is common postpartum.

Breast and Breastfeeding

- Colostrum appears within 12 hours and milk comes in approximately 72 hours after delivery.
- Breasts become engorged by postpartum day 3 or 4 and should subside spontaneously within 24–36 hours.
- Assess breasts for infection, and assess nipples for irritation.
- Encourage the wearing of a bra between feedings.
- Assess for mastitis, abscess, milk plug, thrush, etc.
- Proper positioning of infant (football carry) will minimize soreness.

- Breast shields are used to prevent clothing from rubbing on the nipples.
- Apply moist heat for 5 minutes prior to breastfeeding.
- Use ice compress after each feeding to reduce swelling and discomfort.
- Avoid using baby bottles to prevent "nipple confusion."
- Encourage rest and continuation of feeding or pumping.

Abdomen and Uterus

- The uterus should be firm, about the size of a grapefruit, central, and at the level of the umbilicus immediately postpartum. Deviation to the right may indicate a distended bladder.
- Assess for bladder fullness; have mother void if bladder is full. A full bladder may inhibit uterine contractions, causing bleeding.
- If postvoid uterus is still boggy, massage top of fundus with fingers held together and reassess every 15 minutes.
- Mother and/or partner may be instructed to massage fundus.
- Auscultate bowel sounds and inquire daily about bowel movements.
- Constipation is common from anesthesia and analgesics and from fear of perineal pain.
- Increased fiber and fluid intake, along with early and routine ambulation, will help to reduce the occurrence of constipation.

Perineum

- Episiotomy: assess for swelling, bleeding, stitches, and infection.
- Hemorrhoids: encourage sitz baths to help reduce discomfort.
- Lochia: assess amount, character, and color. Explain the stages and duration of lochia discharge and instruct client to report any odor.
  - **Lochia rubra:** 1–3 days postpartum; mostly blood and clots.
  - **Lochia serosa:** 4–10 days postpartum; serosanguineous.
  - **Lochia alba:** 11–21 days postpartum; creamy white, scant flow.

Lower Extremities

- Thrombophlebitis: unilateral swelling; decreased pulses; redness; heat; tenderness; positive Homan's sign. Leg exercises and early ambulation help minimize venous stasis and clot formation.

Emotional Status

- Explain to the mother and to her family that her emotions may shift from high to low and that these changes are considered normal as a result of the tremendous hormonal changes occurring postpartum.
- Assess parent–infant bonding and family support system.

Newborn Care

Initial Newborn Assessment

Normal Newborn Vital Signs				
	Respirations	Heart Rate	Systolic Blood Pressure	Temperature
Preterm	50–70/min	140–180/min	40–60 mm Hg	36.8°C–37.5°C
Newborn	30–60/min	120–160/min	60–90 mm Hg	36.8°C–37.5°C

Normal Newborn Measurements	
Weight	6–10 lbs
Length	18–22 inches
Head circumference	33–35 cm
Chest circumference	30–33 cm

APGAR Assessment Tool		
Appearance	1 min	5 min
• Pink torso and extremities: 2 • Pink torso, blue extremities: 1 • Blue all over: 0		
Pulse	1 min	5 min
• Greater than 100: 2 • Less than 100: 1 • Absent: 0		
Grimace (irritability)	1 min	5 min
• Vigorous cry: 2 • Limited cry: 1 • No response to stimuli: 0		

Continued

APGAR Assessment Tool—cont'd

Activity	1 min	5 min
• Actively moving: 2 • Limited movement: 1 • Flaccid: 0		
Respiratory effort	**1 min**	**5 min**
• Strong loud cry: 2 • Hypoventilation, irregular: 1 • Absent: 0		
Totals*		

*8–10: normal; 4–6: moderate depression; 0–3: aggressive resuscitation.

Note: Some hospitals require a 10-minute APGAR score.

Initial Newborn Nursing Care

Patent Airway
- Baby should be pink and have a loud, vigorous cry.
- Suction the nose and mouth to clear excess secretions and mucus.
- Insert bulb syringe or DeLee® catheter along side of mouth to avoid gag reflex; use side-lying position with roll behind back.

Body Temperature
- Stimulate breathing with vigorous rubbing and drying.
- Dry baby and maintain warmth (e.g., wrap in blankets, warmer). Put on cap; place on mother's abdomen.
- Cover with warm blanket in an isolette or unclothed under radiant warmer.
- Assess temperature (axillary or aural) every hour until stable. Rectal temperature route is contraindicated.
- Newborn is unable to shiver and breaks down brown fat to produce energy for warmth. Stress increases need for oxygen and upsets acid–base balance.

Identification

- Place ID bands on baby and mother with name, sex, date, time of birth, and ID number.
- Record baby's footprints on form with mother's fingerprints, name, date, and time of birth.
- Identify before mother and newborn are separated.

Eye Prophylaxis

- Apply ophthalmic antibiotic to lower conjunctiva of each eye (prevents gonorrheal or chlamydial infection of eyes contracted during vaginal birth).
- Administer antibiotic after parent–newborn attachment is facilitated.

Vitamin K

- Administer IM dose of vitamin K to promote normal clotting. Vitamin K is produced in the GI tract when bacterial formation occurs after ingesting breast milk or formula, usually by the 8th day.
- **The IM injection is given in the infant's thigh.**

Umbilical Cord

- Clamp for 24 hours or until cord is dry.
- Assess for bleeding or infection.
- Clean cord with soap and water after each diaper change, and apply topical antibiotic if ordered. Place diaper below umbilical cord stump.
- Advise family to continue care until cord falls off (about 10–14 days).

Bathing

- Bathe with warm water and mild soap to remove amniotic fluid, blood, vaginal secretions, and skin residue. Keep environment warm and draft-free to decrease chilling. Dry and swaddle baby.
- Advise family to sponge bathe infant daily and give tub bath after cord falls off and circumcision is healed (usually 2 weeks).

Circumcision

- Assess for swelling, redness, bleeding q30min for 2 hours, then q2h for 24 hours, then with each diaper change.
- Monitor urination (less than six diapers a day may indicate edema is occluding urethra).
- Change dressing as ordered (e.g., three times on first day and then daily for 3 days). Use diaper ointment or petroleum jelly.
- Avoid disrupting yellowish exudate that appears on second day because this is part of the healing process.

- Apply diaper loosely to decrease pressure and friction.
- Administer analgesic as ordered.

Phenylketonuria (PKU)
- The blood sample for PKU screening should be obtained 24 hours after feeding begins.
- The normal serum blood level is less than 4 mg/dL.
- Obtain the sample from a heel stick using a lancet.

Coombs' Test
- Test is done if mother is **Rh-negative**.
- It determines if the mother has formed harmful antibodies against her fetus's RBCs and transferred them to her baby via the placenta.
- Obtain a sample from a heel stick.

Immunizations
- The physician may order the first hepatitis B vaccine to be given soon after birth, prior to discharge.

Pediatrics

Pediatric Assessment

Normal Pediatric Vital Signs				
Age	RR/min	HR/min	Systolic BP	Temp
Preterm	50–70	140–180	40–60	36.8°C–37.5°C
Newborn	30–60	110–120	60–90	36.8°C–37.5°C
6 months	25–35	110–180	85–105	37.5°C
1 year	20–30	80–160	95–105	37.5°C
2 years	20–30	80–130	95–105	37.5°C
4 years	20–30	80–120	95–110	37.5°C
6 years	18–24	75–115	95–110	37.0°C
8 years	18–22	70–110	95–115	37.0°C
10 years	16–20	70–110	95–120	37.0°C
12 years	16–20	60–110	95–125	37.0°C
Adolescent	12–20	60–100	95–135	37.0°C

Pediatric Assessment

- Have the parent hold the child as much as possible during assessment.
- Begin with data collection and assist with physical assessment last; collect data regarding chief complaint, events surrounding current illness, signs and symptoms, immunization history, allergies, medications, past medical history, and current intake and output.
- Establish trust; use a toy or game as a diversion.
- Communicate with child at his or her eye level using age-appropriate language; use child's name frequently.
- Demonstrate procedures on a doll when appropriate.
- Be truthful, especially when explaining painful procedures.
- Save painful procedures until the end of the assessment.
- Be friendly and assertive; do not give a choice when there is none.

Average Height and Weight (50th Percentile)				
Age	**Height**		**Weight**	
	in	cm	lb	kg
Newborn	18	45.7	8	3.6
6 months	26	66	16	7.2
1 year	30	76.2	21	9.5
2 years	34	86.4	27	12.2
4 years	40	101.6	35	16
6 years	45	114.3	45	20.5
8 years	50	127	56	25.5
10 years	55	139.7	73	33.2
12 years	60	152.4	92	41.8
Adolescent	65	165.1	>110	>50

Pediatric Assessment/Growth and Development

Age	Developmental Milestones
1 month	Cries to communicate; reflex activity; eye contact
2 months	Coos; smiles; frowns; tracks objects; lifts head
3 months	Turns from back to side; sits with support
4 months	Turns from back to abdomen; lifts head; bears weight on forearms; can hold head erect; places everything in mouth; grasps with both hands; laughs; makes constant sounds
5 months	Turns from abdomen to back; uses hands independently; plays with toes; puts feet into mouth
6 months	Sits alone leaning forward on hands; holds bottle; extends arms to be picked up; shows fear of strangers; begins to make wordlike sounds; looks for dropped objects; plays "peek-a-boo"
7 months	Sits erect; begins to crawl; bears weight on feet when supported
8 months	Pulls to a standing position; sits alone without support; increased fear of strangers
9 months	Walks holding onto furniture; well-developed crawl; bangs objects together; drinks from cup; attempts to feed self; develops object permanence
10 months	May begin to walk and climb; dominant hand apparent; may say one or two meaningful words
11 months	Understands meaning of "No"; shakes head to indicate "No"; can follow simple directions; cooperates when dressing; uses spoon
12 months	Walks alone or with one hand held; falls frequently while walking; points with one finger; drinks well from cup; pulls off socks; triples birth weight
15 months	Walks independently; throws overhanded; pulls or pushes toys; builds with blocks; scribbles with crayon
18 months	Runs clumsily; jumps in place with both feet; says about 10 words; may have bladder and/or bowel control; anterior fontanel closed

Pediatric Assessment/Growth and Development—cont'd

Age	Developmental Milestones
2 years	Runs well; climbs stairs by placing both feet on each step; attains bladder/bowel control between ages 2 and 3; names familiar objects; combines two to three words
2 ½ years	Jumps from chair or steps; stands on one foot briefly; quadruples birth weight
3 years	Rides tricycle; turns doorknobs; climbs stairs by alternating feet; dresses self; uses short sentences; knows approximately 900 words; increases weight by 5 lbs/year through age 5 (average); increases height by 2.5–3 inches per year thru age 5 (average)
4 years	Hops on one foot; catches ball; names colors; knows approximately 1,500 words
5 years	Skips well; jumps rope; maintains balance with eyes closed; uses complete sentences; vocabulary of approximately 2,100 words; personality has developed; shares with others
6–12 years	Swims; skates; rides bicycle; ties shoes; uses crayon or pencil well; has strong sense of fairness; awareness of rule-governed behavior; uses complex sentences; reads; counts; forms clubs or groups; increases weight by 4.5–6.5 lbs per year (average); increases height by 2 inches per year (average); erupts permanent teeth beginning with front teeth; onset of puberty
12–21 years	Learns to care for self independently while learning to interact with society; puberty in early adolescence (11–14 years); transition to peer group identification in middle adolescence (15–17 years); transitions into adulthood in late adolescence (18–21 years); motivated by peer group; increased interest in sex; capable of abstract, conceptual, and hypothetical thinking

Recommended Immunization Schedule for Ages 0–6 Years

Recommended Immunization Schedule for Persons Aged 0–6 Years   UNITED STATES • 2009

Vaccine ▼ Age ►	Birth	1 month	2 months	4 months	6 months	12 months	15 months	18 months	19–23 months	2–3 years	4–6 years
Hepatitis B	Hep B	Hep B			Hep B						
Rotavirus			RV	RV	RV						
Diptheria, Tetanus, Pertussis			DTaP	DTaP	DTaP		DTaP				DTaP
Haemophilus Influenzae type b			Hib	Hib	Hib	Hib					
Pneumococcal			PCV	PCV	PCV	PCV				PPSV	
Inactivated Poliovirus			IPV	IPV	IPV						IPV
Influenza						Influenza (Yearly)					
Measles, Mumps, Rubella						MMR					MMR
Varicella						Varicella					Varicella
Hepatitis A						HepA (2 doses)				HepA Series	
Meningococcal											MCV

▨ Range of recommended ages   ▮ Certain high-risk groups

Recommended Immunization Schedule for Ages 7–18 Years

Recommended Immunization Schedule for Persons Aged 7–18 Years UNITED STATES · 2009

For those who fall behind or start late, see the schedule below and the catch-up schedule

Vaccine ▼ Age ▶	7–10 years	11–12 years	13–18 years
Diptheria, Tetanus, Pertussis		Tdap	Tdap
Human Papillomavirus		HPV (3 doses)	HPV Series
Meningococcal	MCV	MCV	MCV
Influenza		Influenza (Yearly)	
Pneumococcal		PPSV	
Hepatitis A		HepA Series	
Hepatitis B		HepB Series	
Inactivated Poliovirus		IPV Series	
Measles, Mumps, Rubella		MMR Series	
Varicella		Varicella Series	

- ▮ Range of recommended ages
- ▮ Catch-up immunization
- ▮ Certain high-risk groups

Pediatric Pain Assessment

	Pediatric Pain Assessment
Age	**Signs and Symptoms**
Infant	Grimacing; frowning; startled expression; high-pitched, loud cry; thrashing of extremities; ↑ HR; ↑ BP; ↓ O₂ sats.
Toddler	Guarding; rubbing area; restlessness; loud cry; may verbalize with words such as, "boo boo;" ↑ HR; ↑ BP.
Preschooler	May perceive pain as punishment; may deny pain to avoid treatment; able to describe location and intensity; cries and kicks; may be withdrawn.
School-aged	Fear of bodily harm and mutilation; aware of death; able to describe pain; may have stiff body posture; may withdraw; may attempt to delay procedure.
Adolescent	Perceives pain at physical, emotional, and cognitive levels; able to describe pain; increased muscle tension; may withdraw; may show decreased motor activity.

Pediatric Pain Interventions

Nonopioid Analgesics

■ **Acetaminophen (Tylenol®):** 10–15 mg/kg PO q4h; max. 5 doses daily.
■ **Ibuprofen (Advil®):** >2 years; 7.5 mg/kg PO qid; max. 30 mg/kg daily.
■ **Naproxen sodium (Naprosyn®):** >2 years; 5 mg/kg PO bid; max. 2 doses.
■ **Lidocaine/prilocaine topical (EMLA®):** <5 mg: max. 1 g over 10 cm for 1 hour; 5–10 kg: max. 2 g over 20 cm for 4 hours; 10–20 kg: 10 g over 100 cm for 4 hours; >20 kg: max. 20 g over 200 cm for 4 hours.

Opioid Analgesics

■ **Codeine:** >1 year; 0.5 mg/kg PO, IM, SC q 4–6 hours; max. four doses daily; not recommended for IV use.
■ **Meperidine (Demerol®):** 1.1–1.8 mg/kg PO, IM, SC q 3–4 hours prn; max. 50–100 mg/dose.
■ **Morphine:** 0.1-0.2 mg/kg IV, IM, SC prn; max 15 mg/dose.
■ **Fentanyl citrate (Sublimaze®):** >2 years; 2-3 mcg/kg IV.

Nonpharmacological Interventions

- **Distraction:** Use for mild pain relief.
- **Guided imagery:** Aid the child in creating a pleasurable mental image during the painful situation.
- **Thought stopping:** Stop the painful thought with a positive thought.
- **Soothing music or aromatherapy:** Use to calm emotions and state of mind.
- **Thermotherapy:** Apply warm and cold to painful areas to promote circulation or reduce edema with limited numbing effect.
- **Gentle massage:** Relax or focus child away from pain toward more gentle soothing touch.
- **Sucrose "sweet" nipple:** Calm young infants by allowing them to suck on a bottle nipple dipped in sucrose solution; this is an effective method in reducing pain during procedures.

Pediatric Injection Sites	
Infant	**IM:** Ventrogluteal or vastus lateralis with 5/8-inch to 7/8-inch needle **IV:** 20–24-gauge over-the-needle catheter with burette or infusion device; use scalp veins, dorsal hand, wrist, antecubital site, or feet for infants not yet walking
Toddler	**IM:** Ventrogluteal or dorsogluteal with 5/8-inch to 1-inch needle **IV:** 20–24-gauge over-the-needle catheter with burette or infusion device; use nondominant hand, wrist, or antecubital site
Older child	**IM:** Ventrogluteal or deltoid with 5/8-inch to 1-inch needle **IV:** 20–24-gauge over-the-needle catheter with burette or infusion device; use nondominant hand, wrist, or antecubital site

Common Pediatric Disorders

Constipation

- **Causes:** Transient illness; dietary changes; travel; medications; withholding behaviors (as with painful BMs); overzealous toilet training; emotional stress.
- **Signs/Symptoms:** Distended abdomen; rectal fullness; straining during BM; blood-streaked BMs; decreased bowel sounds.
- **Treatment:** May resolve spontaneously; stool softeners; laxatives; suppositories; enemas; increased fluid and/or fiber intake; mineral oil.
- **Nursing Interventions:**
  - **Rectal stimulation with cotton-tipped applicator or thermometer is contraindicated because of risk of pain and anal fissures.**
  - Collect data related to age of onset, diet, bowel habits, stool frequency, amount, color, and consistency.
  - Teach dietary modifications, such as ↑ fiber, ↑ raw fruit and vegetables; ↑ oral fluids, and bowel training (sitting on toilet for at least 10 minutes at the same time each day).

Diarrhea

- **Causes:**
  - *Acute:* viral, bacterial, and parasitic pathogens; upper respiratory infection; urinary tract infection; antibiotic therapy; laxatives; excess sorbitol or fructose (apple juice and candy); attends day care; recent travel.
  - *Chronic:* malabsorption syndromes; food allergies; inflammatory bowel disease; AIDS.
- **Signs/Symptoms:** Frequent, watery stools; >10% weight loss; increased vital signs; pale, gray, or mottled skin; irritability; lethargy; perianal excoriation.
- **Treatment:** Oral rehydration therapy with glucose/electrolyte solution; 4–8 oz for each diarrheal stool; eliminate or restrict cause; antibiotics for positive stool culture.
- **Nursing Interventions:**
  - If acutely ill with fever, avoid sugary fluids (such as fruit juice, carbonated beverages, and gelatin).
  - Observe for signs and symptoms of dehydration and electrolyte imbalances.

- Collect data related to pattern and duration of diarrhea, amount, and characteristics of stool; vital signs; daily weight; and diarrhea in relation to fluids, food, or medications.
- Change diaper often and apply skin barrier (such as diaper ointment).
- Encourage breastfeeding mother to continue breastfeeding.
- Teach dietary restrictions if ordered.

Dehydration in the Pediatric Client

- **Causes**: Decreased fluid absorption; decreased fluid intake; GI losses from vomiting, diarrhea, or nasogastric suctioning; increased urinary output secondary to diabetes mellitus and inappropriate antidiuretic hormone (ADH) secretion; diaphoresis; fever; ↑ environmental temperature; ↑ activity; hemorrhage.
- **Signs/Symptoms**: Dry mucus membranes; ↓ urine output; irritability; lethargy; pale, gray, or mottled skin; ↓ skin turgor; ↓ blood pressure; ↑ heart rate; ↑ respirations.
- **Treatment**: Oral replacement therapy: 50–100 mL/kg for mild/moderate dehydration; IV fluid replacement for severe dehydration: 1–3 boluses of NS or LR, 20 to 30 mL/kg; maintenance fluids to ↑ extracellular fluid; sodium bicarbonate to correct metabolic acidosis; potassium replacement.
- **Nursing Interventions**:
  - **Rapid fluid replacement is contraindicated with hypertonic dehydration because of risk of water toxicity; potassium should be withheld until kidney function is assessed and circulation improves.**
  - **1 gram wet diaper weight = 1 mL urine.**
  - Administer fluids and electrolytes as ordered.
  - Collect data related to signs and symptoms of dehydration, excess fluids, and urine output.
  - Check vital signs as ordered, monitor I&O, and weigh as ordered.

Nausea and Vomiting (N&V)

- **Causes**: Transient illness; high intestinal obstruction; ↓ gastric emptying; allergies; poisoning; drug toxicity; appendicitis; pancreatitis; peptic ulcer disease; ↑ intracranial pressure; metabolic disorder; hypertrophic pyloric stenosis.
- **Signs/Symptoms**: Salivation; pallor; diaphoresis; ↑ heart rate; green bilious vomiting (bowel obstruction); curdled vomitus (↓ gastric emptying); fever and diarrhea (infection); vomiting with constipation

(GI obstruction); vomiting with abdominal pain (appendicitis, pancreatitis, peptic ulcer); vomiting with ↓ level of consciousness (LOC) (↑ intracranial pressure, metabolic disorder); projectile vomiting (hypertrophic pyloric stenosis, ↑ intracranial pressure).

- **Treatment:** Treat underlying cause; prevent/treat fluid and electrolyte imbalances (oral rehydration therapy/IV fluids); antiemetics; ↑ carbohydrates to spare protein and prevent ketosis.
- **Nursing Interventions:**
  - **Place client in side-lying position with HOB elevated to 30 degrees to prevent aspiration.**
  - Check vital signs as ordered, monitor I&O, and weigh as ordered.
  - Collect data related to pattern and duration of vomiting; amount and characteristics of vomitus; and vomiting in relation to food, medications, or toxic substances.
  - Observe for complications, such as dehydration and fluid/electrolyte imbalances.
  - Provide hygiene after vomiting.
  - Reintroduce fluids/food slowly.

Childhood Illnesses

Cancer

Leukemia
- **Types:**
  - Acute lymphoid leukemia (ALL).
  - Acute myelogenous leukemia (AML).
- **Causes:** Unrestricted proliferation of immature white blood cells.
- **Signs/Symptoms:** ↓ leukocytes; ↓ RBCs; ↓ neutrophils; ↓ platelets; pallor; fatigue; irritability; increased T-cells; anorexia; decreased weight; bleeding tendencies; bone and joint pain; enlarged liver, spleen, and lymph nodes; central nervous system involvement; usually occurs in 2–6-year-olds; onset is insidious to acute.
- **Treatment:** Based on staging; IV and intrathecal chemotherapy given via four-phase protocol to achieve remission; bone marrow transplant.

- ■ **Nursing Interventions:**
  - ▪ Depends on the effects of medication regimen, extent of myelosuppression, and degree of leukemic infiltration.
  - ▪ Handle gently to decrease pain, bleeding, and fractures.
  - ▪ Provide emotional support for child/parents coping with diagnosis of cancer, invasive tests, chronic course, and potential for relapse and death.
  - ▪ Monitor VS (particularly temperature and BP).
  - ▪ Provide balance between rest and quiet play.
  - ▪ Teach infection prevention.
  - ▪ Support child coping with side effects of medications.
  - ▪ Give analgesics as ordered.

Wilms' Tumor (Nephroblastoma)

- ■ **Causes:** Possibly genetic; malignant tumor of kidney; associated with other congenital disorders.
- ■ **Signs/Symptoms:** Presents as nontender, firm mass deep within unilateral flank; fatigue; weight loss; malaise; dyspnea; hematuria; ↑ temperature; ↑ BP; metastasizes to lung, liver, bone and/or brain; usually occurs before age 5.
- ■ **Treatment:** Radiation and/or chemotherapy before and/or after surgery; excision of adrenal gland; affected lymph nodes, and adjacent organs; one kidney excised if unilateral; one kidney excised and partial nephrectomy of less affected kidney if bilateral.
- ■ **Nursing Interventions:**
  - ▪ Depends on treatment regimen and extent of metastasis.
  - ▪ **DO NOT palpate abdomen to prevent dissemination of cancer cells or rupture tumor capsule.**
  - ▪ Monitor VS, particularly temperature and BP.
  - ▪ Teach infection prevention.
  - ▪ Teach turning, coughing, and deep breathing to prevent respiratory problems because operative site is close to diaphragm.
  - ▪ Give analgesics as ordered.
  - ▪ Provide emotional support for child and parents.

Cerebral Palsy

- **Causes:** Multiple causes such as cerebral anoxia, teratogens, brain malformations, intrauterine infections, prematurity, or childhood meningitis.
- **Signs/Symptoms:** Poor head control and failure to smile by 3 months; unable to sit by 8 months; stiff arms/legs; crossed legs (scissoring); floppiness; pushes away or arches back; irritability and crying; persistent primitive reflexes; tongue thrusting and choking after 6 months; walking on toes; ADHD; seizures.
  - *Spastic:* hypertonicity; decreased balance and coordination; decreased fine and gross motor skills.
  - *Ataxic:* wide-based gait; poor performance of rapid repetitive movements or use of upper extremities.
  - *Dyskinetic-athetoid:* abnormal involuntary movements; slow, writhing movements; drooling and imperfect articulation.
- **Treatment:**
  - PT (braces, splints); occupational therapy (OT) (adaptive equipment); speech therapy.
  - Surgery: tendon lengthening; selective dorsal rhizotomy.
  - Medications: skeletal muscle relaxants; antiseizure; botulinum toxin type A.
  - Education: early intervention; individualized education program (IEP).
  - Increased calories for energy expenditure; increased protein for muscle activity; increased vitamin B_6 for amino acid metabolism.
- **Nursing Interventions:**
  - Teach careful eating, safe environment, and helmet use.
  - Do not overstimulate; engage in play appropriate for developmental level/activity.
  - Assist with bowel and bladder training.
  - Provide ROM to stretch heel cords and prevent contractures.
  - Teach health maintenance and rehabilitation.
  - Teach use and care of orthotics, walking aids, and adaptive devices.
  - Teach about side effects of medications.
  - Assist parents and child coping with lifelong disability.

Congenital Heart Defects

Defects With Decreased Pulmonary Blood Flow
Tetralogy of Fallot
- **Causes:** Four congenital defects: pulmonary valve stenosis, ventricular septal defect, overriding aorta, and right ventricular hypertrophy; pathophysiology depends on extent of defects.
- **Signs/Symptoms:** Mild to acute cyanosis; murmur; acute episodes of cyanosis (blue spells) and hypoxia (tet spells) when energy demands exceed O_2 supply (e.g., crying, feeding).

Tricuspid Atresia
- **Causes:** Congenital; absence of tricuspid valve; no communication between right atrium and right ventricle; incompatible with life without connection between right and left sides of heart (e.g., patent foramen ovale, atrial septal defect, patent ductus arteriosis, ventricular septal defect).
- **Signs/Symptoms:** Cyanosis; tachycardia; dyspnea.

Defects With Increased Pulmonary Blood Flow
Atrial Septal Defect
- **Causes:** Congenital; abnormal opening between atria; right atrial and ventricular enlargement stretches conduction fibers causing dysrhythmias.
- **Signs/Symptoms:** Murmur heard high in chest with fixed splitting of second heart sound.

Patent Ductus Arteriosus
- **Causes:** Congenital; continued patency of fetal connection between aorta and pulmonary artery; ↑ atrial and ventricular workload results in ↑ pulmonary vascular congestion.
- **Signs/Symptoms:** Often asymptomatic; machine-type murmur throughout heartbeat in left 2nd or 3rd intercostal space; bounding pulses; widened pulse pressure.

Ventricular Septal Defect
- **Causes:** Congenital; abnormal opening between ventricles; ↑ right ventricular pressure results in pulmonary hypertension and right ventricular hypertrophy.
- **Signs/Symptoms:** Low, harsh murmur heard throughout systole.

Transposition of the Great Vessels

- **Causes:** Congenital; aorta exits from right ventricle and pulmonary artery exits from the left ventricle; no communication between pulmonary and systemic circulation; incompatible with life without connection between right and left sides of the heart (e.g., patent foramen ovale, atrial septal defect, patent ductus arteriosis, ventricular septal defect).
- **Signs/Symptoms:** Mild to severe cyanosis; heart sounds and other signs and symptoms depend on associated defects.

Truncus Arteriosus

- **Causes:** Congenital; blood from ventricles enters single great vessel that arises from base of heart, directing blood to both pulmonary and systemic circulation; more blood flows to pulmonary arteries because of ↓ resistance resulting in hypoxia.
- **Signs/Symptoms:** Systolic murmur; single, semilunar valve produces loud second heart sound that is not split; variable cyanosis; delayed growth; activity intolerance.

Obstructive Defects

Aortic Stenosis

- **Causes:** Congenital; narrowing of the aortic valve resulting in ↓ cardiac output, left ventricular hypertrophy, and ↑ vascular congestion.
- **Signs/Symptoms:** Murmur; faint pulses; ↓ BP; tachycardia; poor feeding; exercise intolerance.

Coarctation of the Aorta

- **Causes:** Congenital; narrowing of aorta near insertion of ductus arteriosis resulting in ↑ pressure proximal to defect and ↓ pressure distal to defect.
- **Signs/Symptoms:** ↑ BP; bounding radial/carotid pulses; ↓ BP in lower extremities; weak or absent femoral pulses; lower extremities cool to touch.

Pulmonic Stenosis

- **Causes:** Congenital; narrowing of the pulmonary valve; ↓ pulmonary blood flow; right ventricular hypertrophy.
- **Signs/Symptoms:** Murmur; mild cyanosis; cardiomegaly; often asymptomatic.

Nursing Interventions for Congenital Heart Defects

- Assess for S&S specific to disorder, hypoxia, pulmonary congestion, systemic venous congestion, and HF.
- Monitor VS, heart and breath sounds, pulse oximetry, ECG; I&O, and daily weight.
- Maintain fluid restriction if ordered.
- Administer electrolytes, especially for hypokalemia (decreased BP, irritability, decreased pulse, drowsiness, increased risk for digoxin toxicity).
- Facilitate breathing (elevate HOB 30-45 degrees); avoid constipation and constrictive clothing.
- Administer oxygen if ordered.
- Manage hypercyanotic spells by soothing if crying; hold in knee–chest position with head elevated.
- Facilitate feeding (small feedings q2–3 hr, soft nipple with large hole to decrease work of sucking, burp frequently, provide gavage feedings if ordered).
- Prepare for surgery.
- Support parents, discuss specifics of disorder and appropriate care, decrease overdependency by child, and encourage delegation to prevent parental exhaustion.

Complications of Congenital Heart Defects

Heart Failure (HF)

- Heart unable to pump enough blood to meet body's metabolic demands because of decreased myocardial contractility, increased volume of blood returning to heart, and increased resistance against blood being ejected from left ventricle.
- **Signs/Symptoms:** Increased pulse; weak peripheral pulses; decreased BP; gallop rhythm; diaphoresis; decreased urinary output; pale, cool extremities; fatigue; restlessness; weakness; anorexia.

Pulmonary Congestion

- Excessive amount of blood in pulmonary vascular bed; pulmonary edema; associated with left-sided HF.
- **Signs/Symptoms:** Increased pulse; dyspnea; retractions in infants; flaring nares; wheezing; grunting; cyanosis; cough; hoarseness; orthopnea; activity intolerance.

Systemic Venous Congestion

- Increased pressure and pooling of blood in venous circulation; called cor pulmonale if there is a primary lung disease (e.g., cystic fibrosis).
- **Signs/Symptoms:** Increased weight; peripheral and periorbital edema; hepatomegaly; ascites; distended neck veins in children.

Cystic Fibrosis

- **Causes:** Autosomal recessive disease; causes ↑ viscosity of mucus from exocrine glands and abnormal glandular secretion of ions; autosomal recessive disease.
- **Signs/Symptoms:** Variable; may be asymptomatic for months or years; suspected with meconium ileus, failure to regain weight loss at birth, and failure to thrive; frequent RTIs; nonproductive cough; wheezing; chest x-ray shows atelectasis and emphysema; pulmonary function tests reveal small airway dysfunction; foul-smelling, pale, bulky, watery stools; stools contain high fat content and pancreatic enzymes.
  - *Chronic signs/symptoms:* decreased salivation, paroxysmal cough, dyspnea, cyanosis, barrel chest, distended abdomen, thin extremities, clubbing of fingers/toes, rectal prolapse, F&E imbalances, bruising resulting from decreased vitamin K.
- **Treatment:** Oral fluids and medication (Pulmozyme®) to decrease mucus viscosity; chest PT; bronchodilators; antiinflammatories; antibiotics; increased protein and increased calorie diet; salt supplements prn; pancreatic enzymes with meals and snacks to decrease steatorrhea and increase growth; vitamins A, D, E, and K; daily aerobic exercise; lung transplant.
- **Nursing Interventions:**
  - Respiratory functioning:
    - Observe for S&S of respiratory distress; balance rest/activity.
    - Increase fluids to decrease mucus viscosity.
    - Teach how to increase expectoration.
  - GI functioning:
    - Monitor weight, abdominal distention, and stools for characterics and frequency.
    - Monitor for S&S of intestinal obstruction.
    - Teach to increase protein and increase calories.
    - Give pancreatic enzymes with food.

- Ensure adequate salt intake; particularly in hot weather.
- Use perineal skin barrier to protect skin from GI enzymes.
- Psychosocial support:
  - Provide age-appropriate support to increase coping with chronic illness, respiratory equipment, invasive procedures, and infertility/sterility.
  - Promote a positive self-image.
- Parents:
  - Assist parents with shock and guilt, chronicity of illness, and potential for death.
  - Reinforce teaching of chest PT and perform daily in AM and PM; perform between meals to prevent vomiting.
  - Teach diaphragmatic breathing and coughing.
  - Encourage support of child's independence and limit overindulgence to decrease secondary gains.
  - Ensure routine immunizations and flu vaccine at 6 months and then yearly.
  - Refer to genetic counseling and the Cystic Fibrosis Foundation.

Effects of Cystic Fibrosis on Other Organ Systems

Respiratory	Mucus obstructs respiratory passages; mucus stagnation causes hypercapnea, hypoxia, acidosis, and infection; increased lung dysfunction causes emphysema, cor pulmonale, respiratory failure, and death.
Pancreas	Decreased secretion of chloride and bicarbonate; mucus blocks enzymes for reaching duodenum; fibrosis may result in diabetes mellitus.
Liver	Local biliary obstruction and fibrosis results in biliary cirrhosis.
Reproductive	Delayed puberty; females may be infertile; males usually sterile as a result of mucus blocking system.
Integument	Increased secretion of sodium and chloride in saliva and sweat; hyperthermic conditions; dehydration.

Diabetes Mellitus (DM) in Children

Nursing care for diabetes mellitus can be found in Tab 5—Medical/
Surgical Nursing

Gastrointestinal Disorders

Cleft Lip and Cleft Palate

- **Cleft lip:** Unilateral or bilateral fissure in lip; more common in boys.
- **Cleft palate:** Unilateral or bilateral, complete or incomplete opening in
  soft and/or hard palate; may include lip; more common in girls.
- **Causes:** Genetic aberration or teratogens (drugs, viruses, other toxins).
- **Signs/Symptoms:** Difficulty in feeding (decreased ability to form
  vacuum with mouth; may be able to breastfeed); mouth breathing
  with increased swallowed air, which distends abdomen and dries
  mucous membranes; recurrent otitis media; decreased hearing from
  inefficient Eustachian tubes; impaired speech secondary to inefficient
  muscles from malformed soft palate and nasopharynx; decreased
  hearing; misaligned teeth.
- **Treatment:** Surgical repair; possible follow-up with speech therapists
  and orthodontists.
- **Nursing Interventions:**

Preoperative:

- Prevent aspiration (feed with HOB elevated, place nipple in back
  of oral cavity or deposit formula gradually on back of tongue via
  feeding device).
- Burp frequently; place in partial side-lying position with elevated
  HOB; gently suction oropharynx as needed.

Postoperative:

- Prevent aspiration.
- Prevent trauma to suture line by limiting crying, if possible, and
  maintaining position of lip-protective device.
- Use elbow restraints if necessary; place on back/side-lying or in
  infant seat.
- Cleanse suture line after each feeding.

- Assess for increased swallowing that may indicate bleeding.
- Give analgesic, sedative, or antibiotic as ordered.
- Help parents express feelings; show pictures of successful repairs; teach preoperative and postoperative care; encourage cuddling.

Colic

- **Causes:** Immature nervous system; cow's milk allergy; excessive swallowing of air; diet of breastfeeding mother; secondhand smoke.
- **Signs/Symptoms:** Inconsolable, loud crying; legs pulled up to abdomen >3 hours per day for >3 days per week; tense, distended abdomen; ↑ flatus.
- **Treatment:** Rule out other causes of infant distress; treat symptomatically.
- **Nursing Interventions:**
  - Collect data regarding frequency, duration, and characteristics of crying and relationship between crying and feedings; infant's diet; breastfeeding mother's diet; stooling and voiding patterns; sleep patterns; environmental stimuli; behaviors of caregivers.
  - Change modifiable factors that may contribute to abdominal pain.
  - Implement **5 Ss:**
    - **S**waddle tightly in receiving blanket
    - **S**ucking (pacifier, mother's nipple)
    - **S**ide/**S**tomach lying with monitoring
    - **S**hushing sounds (white noise, machine, or CD)
    - **S**winging (rhythmic movements with bed vibrator, swing)
  - Teach proper feeding techniques; eliminate secondhand smoke.
  - Apply pressure to abdomen; massage abdomen.
  - Maintain calm environment; encourage parents to seek respite from child care.

Nasopharyngeal and Tracheoesophageal Anomalies

- **Choanal atresia:** Lack of opening between one or both nasal passages and nasopharynx.
- **Calasia:** Incompetent cardiac sphincter.
- **Esophageal atresia:** Failed esophageal development.
- **Tracheoesophageal fistula:** Opening between trachea and esophagus.
- **Causes:** Genetic aberration or teratogens (drugs, viruses, toxins).

- **Signs/Symptoms:** 3 Cs (coughing, choking, cyanosis) during feeding; excessive salivation and drooling; respiratory distress; abdominal distress; inability to pass a nasogastric tube (NGT).
- **Treatment:** Surgical repair.
- **Nursing Interventions:**

Preoperative:

- Maintain nothing by mouth (NPO).
- Maintain supine and elevated HOB.
- Provide IV fluids.
- Maintain suction of catheter in esophageal pouch as ordered
- Monitor I&O and pulse oximetry.
- Suction oropharynx prn.
- Administer antibiotics as ordered.

Postoperative:

- Maintain airway; monitor I&O, pulse oximetry, and daily weight.
- Administer analgesics and antibiotics as ordered.
- Administer gastrostomy feedings until able to tolerate oral feedings.
- Provide mouth care.
- Change position frequently to prevent pneumonia.
- Provide care of chest tube if present.
- Hold, cuddle, and provide pacifier for nonnutritive sucking.

Hypertrophic Pyloric Stenosis

- **Causes:** Genetic; thickened muscle of pyloric sphincter narrows or obstructs opening between stomach and duodenum; presents 1 to 10 weeks after birth.
- **Signs/Symptoms:** Palpable olive-shaped mass just to right of umbilicus; visible peristaltic waves across abdomen; colicky pain; projectile vomiting; constipation; distention of epigastrum; dehydration; failure to thrive; metabolic acidosis.
- **Treatment:** Surgical repair.
- **Nursing Interventions:**

Preoperative:

- Maintain nothing by mouth (NPO).
- Provide IV fluids to rehydrate and electrolytes to correct imbalances.
- Nasogastric tube to decompress stomach.

Postoperative:

- Begin small, frequent feedings of glucose, water, or electrolyte solution 4–6 hours after surgery and then formula 24 hours later.
- Increase amount and intervals between feedings gradually.

Obstructions

- **Intussusception:** Proximal segment of bowel telescopes into a distal segment; often ileocecal valve; presents at 3–12 months; requires nonsurgical hydrostatic reduction or repair.
- **Volvulus:** Intestine twists around itself; presents during first 6 months; linked to macrorotation of intestine; requires surgical repair.
- **Causes:** Genetic; thickened muscle of pyloric sphincter narrows or obstructs opening between stomach and duodenum; presents 1–10 weeks after birth.
- **Signs/Symptoms:**
  - Intussusception triad:
    - Acute onset to severe paroxysmal abdominal pain.
    - Palpable sausage-shaped mass.
    - Currant jelly stools.
  - Inconsolable crying, kicking, and drawing legs up to abdomen; grunting respirations as a result of abdominal distention; vomiting; lethargy, if untreated; necrosis; perforation; peritonitis; sepsis.
- **Treatment:** Surgical repair or hydrostatic reduction (intussusception).
- **Nursing Interventions:**

Preoperative:

- Maintain NPO status.
- Give analgesics and antibiotics as ordered.

Postoperative:

- Give IV fluids.
- Assess VS and amount and characteristics of stool.
- Assess passage of contrast material if hydrostatic reduction is used for intussusception.
- Give oral feedings as ordered (breastfeeding encouraged to decrease constipation).
- Encourage parental visits.

Exstrophy of the Bladder

- **Causes:** Genetic; absence of a portion of abdominal and bladder wall causing eversion of bladder through opening.
- **Signs/Symptoms:** Leaking of urine; urine smell secondary to leaking; pubic bone malformation; inguinal hernia; epispadias, undescended testes, or short penis in males; cleft clitoris or absent vagina in females.
- **Treatment:** Surgical repair.
- **Nursing Interventions:**

Infant

- Cover bladder with clear plastic wrap or thin film dressing without adhesive.
- Apply prescribed protective barrier to protect skin from urine.
- Monitor I&O and drainage from bladder or ureteral drainage tubes.
- Monitor bowel function if surgery included resection of intestine.
- Care after surgery for penile lengthening, chordee release, and urethral reconstruction similar to hypospadias repair.

Child/Adolescent

- Encourage ventilation of feelings regarding appearance of genitalia, rejection by peers, and ability to function sexually and procreate.
- Care for permanent urinary diversion if present.

Parents

- Support parents coping with child with a defect, multistage surgeries, possible need for permanent urinary diversion, and impact on child's future sexual functioning.
- Teach care of child, including S&S of infection.
- Use clean intermittent catheterization to empty urinary reservoir.

Cryptorchidism (Cryptorchism)

- **Causes:** Genetic; failure of one or both testes to descend into scrotum; increased risk for testicular cancer.
- **Signs/Symptoms:** Nonpalpable testes; affected hemiscrotum appears smaller.

- **Treatment:** Orchiopexy at 6–24 months to prevent torsion (infertility from exposure of testes to body heat).
- **Nursing Interventions:**
  - Monitor urinary functioning and I&O.
  - Prevent contamination of operative site by urine and feces.
  - Apply cool compresses to operative site if ordered.
  - Administer analgesics and antibiotics as ordered.
  - Teach parents to assess testes and scrotum monthly and to teach procedure to child when older.

Displaced Ureteral Openings

- **Hypospadias:** Female has opening in vagina; male has opening on lower surface of penis.
- **Epispadias:** Occurs only in males; opening on dorsal side of penis.
- **Causes:** Genetic; abnormal location of urethral opening.
- **Signs/Symptoms:** Related defects (estrophy of bladder, undescended testes, short penis).
- **Treatment:** Circumcision delayed to preserve tissue; surgical repair.
- **Nursing Interventions:**

Postoperative hypospadias:

  - Assess for S&S of infection.
  - Provide care for indwelling catheter or stent and irrigate if ordered.
  - Avoid tub baths until stent is removed.
  - Apply antibacterial ointment to penis daily.
  - Administer sedatives, analgesics, and antibiotics as ordered.

Postoperative epispadias (see Estrophy of Bladder):

  - Support parents coping with child with a defect, multiple surgeries, and impact on child's future sexual functioning.
  - Teach S&S of infection.
  - Teach care of indwelling catheter (avoid kinks in catheter, never clamp catheter, use urine-collection device in older child to promote mobility).
  - Increase fluid intake.
  - Avoid straddle toys, sandboxes, swimming, and contact sports until permitted.

Inborn Errors of Metabolism

Galactosemia

- **Causes:** Genetic; ↓ carbohydrate metabolism as a result of missing enzyme that converts galactose to glucose.
- **Signs/Symptoms:** Vomiting; S&S of dehydration; malnutrition (decreased weight, muscle mass, and fat); hepatosplenomegaly; jaundice.
- **Treatment:** Elimination of breast milk and foods with milk/lactose; soy-protein formula; dietary restriction for life or relaxed as child develops.
- **Nursing Interventions:**
    - Ensure neonatal screening (Beutler test) is done, particularly for infants born preterm or in the home who were or discharged early.
    - Identify S&S early because treatment prevents or decreases mental retardation.
    - Encourage adherence to drug regimen.
    - Encourage parents and older child to discuss feelings.
    - Refer to dietary counseling and genetic counseling because of genetic transmission.
    - Encourage lifelong medical care.

Phenylketonuria (PKU)

- **Causes:** Genetic; lack of the enzyme that changes phenylalanine into tyrosine.
- **Signs/Symptoms:** Failure to thrive; vomiting; irritability; hyperactivity.
- **Treatment:** Decreased phenylalanine diet to meet growth needs but prevent mental retardation; avoidance of high-protein foods (meat and dairy); diet including most vegetables, fruit, bread, starches, and milk substitutes; total or partial breastfeeding because breast milk has decreased phenylalanine; dietary restrictions are lifelong, particularly before and during pregnancy.
- **Nursing Interventions:** Same as for galactosemia.

Infections and Infestations

Bacterial Meningitis
- **Causes:**
  - *Neonates:* premature rupture of membranes; maternal infection during last week of pregnancy; immune deficiencies.
  - *Children:* bacterial infection; neurosurgical procedures; neurological injuries; chronic diseases; immunosuppression.
- **Signs/Symptoms:** Depend on organism and age; poor feeding; nausea and vomiting; diarrhea; irritability; drowsiness; headache; respiratory irregularities; increased intracranial pressure (ICP).
  - *Neonates:* Increased pitched cry, poor sucking, decreased muscle tone, seizures, bulging fontanels.
  - *Children:* Increased **temperature**, chills, agitation, hallucinations, resistance of neck flexion or hyperextension, photophobia, cyanosis.
- **Treatment:** Initially broad-spectrum antibiotic; specific antibiotic after culture and sensitivity; dexamethasone to decrease ICP; fluids and electrolytes to restore circulating volume; antiepileptic; acetaminophen with codeine for pain.
- **Nursing Interventions:**
  - Encourage flu and pneumococcal vaccination for prevention.
  - Maintain transmission-based precautions for 24–72 hours.
  - Monitor VS, I&O, S&S of increased ICP, neurological status, Glasgow coma scale, and impending shock or seizures.
  - Minimize noise, lights, and touching.
  - Maintain in side-lying position with slight increase in HOB.
  - Provide IV fluids and electrolytes.
  - Provide medications and diet as ordered.
  - Support during frightening procedures.
  - Support parents as they confront the sudden onset of a serious disease.

Candidiasis (Moniliasis)
- **Causes:** *Candida albicans*; infection of skin and/or mucous membranes.
- **Signs/Symptoms:**
  - *Oral lesions:* painless, discrete, bluish-white pseudomembranous patches on oral/pharyngeal mucosa and tongue.
  - *Skin lesions:* scaly, erythematous skin rash, possibly covered with exudates; painful.

- **Treatment:** Antifungals (oral or topical fluconazole preparations); amphotericin B.
- **Nursing Interventions:**
  - Teach hand washing and hygiene.
  - Teach Swedish and swallow technique.

Diaper dermatitis:

- Use superabsorbent disposable diapers and change often.
- Expose skin to air several times a day; apply protective ointment.

Impetigo

- **Causes:** *Staphylococcus* or *Streptococcus* infection of skin; may be superimposed on eczema.
- **Signs/Symptoms:** Reddish macule becomes vesicular and ruptures, leaving superficial, moist erosion; spreads in marginated irregular shapes; lesions dry as honey-colored crusts; pruritis; contagious.
- **Treatment:** Removal of undermined skin, crusts, and debris; topical application of bactericidal ointment; systemic antibiotics.
- **Nursing Interventions:**
  - Teach parents hand washing and about contact isolation, preventing scratching administering medications, and gently rubbing lesions to remove crusts before topical antibiotic application.

Pediculosis (Lice)

- **Causes:** Infestation of head, body, or pubic hair by lice; spread by affected personal articles such as combs, hats, and bedding.
- **Signs/Symptoms:** White eggs (nits) attach to base of hair shafts behind ears and at nape of neck; intense pruritis as a result of crawling insect and insect saliva; papules as a result of secondary infections.
- **Treatment:** Application of pediculicide cream rinse; nit removal with fine-tooth comb.
- **Nursing Interventions:**
  - Wear gloves to apply pediculicide; have child's head over sink, in back-lying position with eyes covered.
  - Remove all visible nits with nit comb.
  - Wash all clothing, bedding, towels in hot water and hot dryer; dry clean unwashables.
  - Vacuum rugs, floors, and furniture.
  - Soak brushes, combs, hats, and scarves in pediculicide for 1 hour.

Ringworm

- **Causes:** Fungal infection.
  - *Tinea capitis:* infection of scalp.
  - *Tinea cruris (jock itch):* infection of thigh, crural fold, and scrotum of men.
  - *Tinea pedis:* infection between toes and on plantar surface of feet.
- **Signs/Symptoms:** Pruritis, characteristic lesions.
  - *Tinea capitis:* patchy, scaly areas of alopecia on scalp; may extend to hairline/neck.
  - *Tinea cruris:* round or oval erythematous scaling patch that spreads peripherally.
  - *Tinea pedis:* maceration and fissuring between toes; pinhead-size vesicles on plantar surface of feet.
- **Treatment:** Oral griseofulvin; local application of antifungal; selenium shampoos for tinea capitis.
- **Nursing Interventions:**
  - Teach personal hygiene.
  - Advise to avoid pets, particularly cats.
  - Advise not to share personal items.
  - Encourage wearing plastic shoes in swimming areas and locker rooms.
  - Encourage wearing cotton socks and underwear and ventilated shoes to decrease heat and perspiration.

Scabies

- **Causes:** Infestation of scabies mites; burrows into and multiplies in epidermis; transmitted by direct contact with infected person.
- **Signs/Symptoms:** Inflammatory response: papules, vesicles, and pustules usually involving hands, wrists, axillae, genitalia, and inner thighs or feet and ankles of children younger than age 2 years; intense itching; mite appears as black dot at end of linear, grayish-brown, threadlike burrow.
- **Treatment:** Application of a topical scabicide or ivermectin tablets; antibiotics for secondary infections.
- **Nursing Interventions:**
  - Advise all in contact with infected person to be treated (time between infestation and S&S is 1–2 months).
  - Thoroughly massage cream into skin surfaces from head to under feet; keep on 8–14 hours; remove by shampooing and bathing.

- Explain that pruritis may take 2–3 weeks to subside.
- After treatment, all linen and contaminated clothing must be washed and dried at high heat settings.

Neurological Disorders

Attention Deficit/Hyperactivity Disorder (ADHD)

- **Causes:** Genetic; slightly smaller brain volume; decreased dopamine level; decreased frontal lobe functioning.
- **Signs/Symptoms:** Characterized by persistent inattention or by hyperactivity/impulsivity for at least 6 months.
  - *Inattention:* includes carelessness and inattention to detail; cannot sustain attention; does not appear to be listening; does not follow through with instructions; unable to finish tasks; difficulty with organization; dislikes activities that require concentration and sustained effort; loses things; distracted by extraneous stimuli; forgetful.
  - *Hyperactivity:* Fidgeting, moving feet, squirming; leaves seat before being excused; runs about/climbs excessively; difficulty playing quietly; described as "on the go" and "driven by a motor;" excessive talking.
  - *Impulsivity:* Blurts out answers; speaks before thinking; problem waiting his or her turn; interrupts or intrudes; impairment is present before age 7.
- **Treatment:**
  - *Nonpharmacological ADHD treatments:* individual/family therapy; set clear expectations and limits; break commands up into clear steps; support desired behaviors and immediately respond to undesired behaviors with consequences; time out may be needed for cooling down/reflecting; role-playing helpful in teaching friend–friend interactions; help child prepare for interactions and understand how intrusive behaviors annoy and drive friends away; important that school knows about ADHD diagnosis; seek out special education services; sit near teacher; one assignment at a time; written instructions; untimed tests, tutoring.
  - *Pharmacological ADHD treatments:* norepinephrine reuptake inhibitors (Strattera®); psychostimulant medications; bupropion (Wellbutrin®); clonidine (Catapres®).

Hydrocephalus

- **Causes:** Abnormal increase of cerebrospinal fluid in ventricular system.
  - *Communicating hydrocephalus:* ↓ absorption of cerebrospinal fluid (CSF) within the subarachnoid space; often as a result of infection, trauma, or thick arachnoid membranes or meninges
  - *Noncommunicating hydrocephalus:* obstruction of flow of CSF through ventricular system; usually as a result of neoplasm, hematoma, or congenital Chiari malformation (herniation of medulla through foramen magnum).
- **Signs/Symptoms:** Increased head size in infant as a result of open sutures/bulging fontanels; sclera visible above iris; retinal papilledema; prominent scalp veins; shiny, taut skin; head lag after 4–6 months of age; may exhibit attention deficit, hyperactivity, mental retardation.
- **Signs/Symptoms of Increased Intracranial Pressure:**
  - *Infant:* projectile vomiting unassociated with feeding; altered feeding behaviors; irritability; increased shrill cry; seizures.
  - *Older child:* headache (usually in the morning); confusion; apathy; decreased LOC.
- **Treatment:** Surgical removal of obstruction; decreasing excessive CSF by shunting fluid out of the ventricles and to the peritoneum; shunt revision as child grows.
- **Nursing Interventions:**

Preoperative:

- Maintain in Fowler's position to help drain CSF.
- Monitor VS.
- Take measurements of head circumferences.
- Assess fontanels for bulging daily.
- Assess for S&S of increased intracranial pressure.
- Support head and neck when holding or moving infant.
- Protect from skin breakdown.
- Keeps eyes moist and free from irritation.
- Provide small, frequent feedings and schedule care around feedings to decrease vomiting.

Postoperative:

- Place on nonoperative side to decrease pressure on shunt; keep flat to prevent rapid ↓ of intracranial fluid that may lead to subdural hematoma.
- Monitor for S&S of infection (shunt malfunction, fever, wound or shunt tract inflammation, poor feeding, vomiting, abdominal pain); most common complication 1–2 months postoperative.

Intellectual Disability

- Types:
  - *Mild:* IQ 50–70; educable; mental age 8–12 years; simple reading, writing, math skills; may function in society and have a job.
  - *Moderate:* IQ 35–55; trainable; mental age 3–7 years; performs ADLs; has social skills; can work in sheltered workshop.
  - *Severe:* IQ 20–40; barely trainable; mental age 2 years; requires supportive, long-term care.
  - *Profound:* IQ <25; mental age <1 year; requires long-term total care.
- **Causes:** Genetic: Down syndrome and Fragile X syndrome; prenatal drug/alcohol use; maternal infections; low folic acid; prematurity; anoxia; cranial malformations; meningitis; measles; lead poisoning.
- **Signs/Symptoms:** Decreased functioning in more than two areas (communication, self-care, home living, social or interpersonal skills, self-direction, functional academic skills); decreased eye contact, decreased spontaneous activity, nonresponsive to contact; delayed developmental milestones; poor results on standardized tests; passive and dependent to aggressive and impulsive; additional problems, such as decreased coordination, motor, hearing, and vision; may have seizures, attention deficit/hyperactivity disorder, or mood disorders.
- **Treatment:** Early identification; early intervention programs; individualized education plans, PT, OT, and vocational therapy (VT); placement in day care, respite program, or long-term care facility.
- **Nursing Interventions:**
  - Use simple, concrete communication and a variety of senses.
  - Teach tasks step-by-step while slowly removing assistance.
  - Give positive reinforcement for desired behavior.
  - Role-play social behaviors; support independence with ADLs; base play on developmental, not chronological, age.
  - Encourage time with peer groups.

- Explore sexuality issues with parents and client.
- Support parents coping with diagnosis and decision concerning temporary/permanent placement.

Neural Tube Defects

- **Types:**
  - *Spina bifida occulta:* defect of vertebrae with intact spinal cord and meninges
  - *Spina bifida cystica:* saclike protrusion on back; the two most common types:
    - *Meningocoele:* the exposed sac contains meninges and spinal fluid.
    - *Myeolmeningocoele:* the sac contains the spinal cord, nerve roots, spinal fluid, and meninges; associated with malformations (intestinal, cardiac, renal, urinary, and orthopedic).
- **Causes:** Congenital defect.
- **Signs/Symptoms:**

Spina bifida occulta:

- May not be visible or may have superficial signs in lumbrosacral area; progressive disturbances of gait; decreased bowel and bladder control.

Spina bifida cystica:

- Vary; depend on anatomic level and extent of defect.
- Sensory disturbances parallel motor impairments.
- Joint deformities as a result of denervation to lower extremities; includes flexion/extension contractures.

Defect below 2nd lumbar vertebrae:

- Flaccid, partial paralysis of legs; varying degrees of decreased sensation; continuous dribbling of urine and overflow incontinence; no bowel control and possible rectal prolapse

Defect below 3rd sacral vertebrae:

- No motor impairment; decreased bowel and bladder control.
- **Treatment:** Surgery within 24–72 hours decreases stretching of nerve roots and lowers risk for trauma to sac, hydrocephalus, and infection.

Eventually artificial sphincters and reservoirs may be created surgically.

- **Nursing Interventions:**
  - Prevent trauma to sac; keep infant naked in radiant warmer.

Preoperative:

- Keep infant prone even when feeding.

Postoperative

- Place infant in prone or partial side-lying position.
- Use sterile, moist, nonadherent dressing to surgical area to decrease drying; change every 2–4 hours.
- Assess for S&S of infection.
- Assess for leaks, tears, and abrasions.
- Keep area free of urine and feces.
- Monitor for hydrocephalus and increased ICP.
- Keep hips in slight abduction; perform PROM to knees, ankles, and feet as ordered.

Child:

- For older child, use braces, walking devices, or wheelchair as ordered.
- Incontinence is most stressful for child's social development; teach clean intermittent catheterization.

Parents:

- Support coping with feelings and decision regarding abortion if identified in utero lifelong care of infant with multiple neurological, genitourinary, and musculoskeletal problems.
- Involve in child's care.
- Refer to support group.

Poisoning

Hydrocarbons

- Kerosene, gasoline, turpentine, furniture polish, cleaning fluids
- **Signs/Symptoms:** Coughing; gagging; nausea and vomiting; lethargy; tachypnea; cyanosis; substernal retractions; grunting.
- **Treatment:** Gastric lavage with endotracheal tube to prevent aspiration; IV fluids; O_2.

Corrosive Chemicals

- Bleach, oven or drain cleaners, detergents, and electric dishwasher granules.
- **Signs/Symptoms:** Severe burning in oral cavity and stomach; white, swollen mucous membranes; edema of lips, tongue, and pharynx; vomiting; hemoptosis; hematemesis; anxiety; agitation.
- **Treatment:** NPO; IV fluids; analgesics; O$_2$; endotracheal tube as needed; repeated dilation or surgery for esophageal stricture.

Lead

- Found in paints, soil, dust, and drinking water.
- **Signs/Symptoms:** Blood concentration >10 mg/100 mL; anemia; lead line on teeth and long bones; joint pain; headache; proteinuria; lethargy; irritability; hyperactivity; insomnia; seizures.
- **Treatment:** Chelation when blood lead levels near 45 μg/dL.

Acetaminophen

- Most common medication poisoning in children.
- **Signs/Symptoms:** History of 150 mg/kg for several days; nausea and vomiting; diaphoresis; ↓ urine output; pallor; weakness; bradycardia; liver failure; RUQ pain; coagulation abnormalities; jaundice; confusion; coma.
- **Treatment:** If ingestion occurred within previous hour, activated charcoal may be given; if longer, administer acetylcysteine (antidote); PO and IV fluids.

Salicylate (ASA)

- **Signs/Symptoms:**

Toxicity:

- ***Acute:*** 300 to 500 mg/kg/day.
- *Chronic:* >100 mg/kg/day
  - Diaphoresis; nausea and vomiting; oliguria; elevated temperature; hyperpnea; tinnitus; dizziness; delirium.

Poisoning: confusion; metabolic acidosis; hyperventilation; coma

- **Treatment:** Gastric lavage; activated charcoal; saline cathartics; intravenous fluids; vitamin K if bleeding; peritoneal dialysis prn; hypothermia blanket prn.
- **Nursing Interventions:**

Emergency care:

- Do not induce vomiting (may redamage mucosa).
- Identify agent; terminate exposure.
- Prevent aspiration; flush eyes/skin with water.
- Transport for medical care and bring evidence (container, vomitus).

Acute care:

- Maintain airway; monitor VS; assess hepatic and renal function.
- Be calm; do not admonish child or parent.

Prevention:

- Teach child not to eat nonfood items (pica) and to follow parents' safety rules.
- Teach parents to keep toxins and drugs in locked cabinet and to use childproof containers.

Respiratory Disorders

Nursing care for the person with respiratory tract infections can be found in Tab 5—Medical/Surgical Nursing.

Signs and Symptoms

- **Laryngitis:** Hoarseness.
- **Tonsillitis:** Tonsils covered with exudate.
- **Epiglottis:** Large cherry-red edematous epiglottis; slow, quiet breathing; no spontaneous cough; agitation; drooling; sore throat.
- **Otitis media:** Pulling at ears or rolling head side to side; earache; sucking or chewing increases pain; bulging red ear drum; may exhibit hearing loss, vomiting, and diarrhea.
- **Laryngotracheobronchitis (Croup):**
  - *Stage I:* fear, hoarseness, barking cough, inspiratory stridor.
  - *Stage II:* dyspnea, retractions; use of accessory muscles.
  - *Stage III:* restlessness; pallor; diaphoresis; increased respirations; S&S of hypoxia; CO_2 retention.
  - *Stage IV:* cyanosis; cessation of breathing

Specific Treatments

- Antibiotics for bacterial infections; rifampin may be added to eliminate group A beta-hemolytic streptococcus.
- Removal of tonsils and adenoids that obstruct breathing or for recurrent infections.
- Antibiotic eardrops, local heat, and myringotomy for otitis media with persistent effusion or hearing loss.
- Corticosteroids; endotracheal intubation or tracheostomy for epiglottis with severe respiratory distress.
- Corticosteroids and nebulized epinephrine for croup.
- Ribavirin for RSV.

Skeletal Disorders

Clubfoot

- **Signs/Symptoms:** Affected foot/feet smaller and shorter with empty heel pad and transverse plantar crease; unilateral affected extremity may be shorter and have calf atrophy; increased risk of hip dysplasia.
- **Treatment:** Serial casts or surgical correction.
- **Nursing Interventions:**
  - Ensure that casts are reapplied as child grows; infant with clubfoot: daily for 2 weeks and then q1–2 weeks for a total of 8–12 weeks.
  - Ensure that splint is applied correctly; splint permits some mobility but prevents hip extension and adduction; straps should be checked q 1–2 weeks and should be worn continuously (3–5 months).
  - Perform neurovascular check (blanching, warm toes, able to move toes, pedal pulse).
  - Cast care: place diaper under edge of cast; transparent film dressing should form bridge between cast and skin; apply clothing over cast to prevent child from stuffing food or objects down cast; assess for odor.
  - Splint care: sponge bathe; keep straps dry; place diaper under straps; dress in knee socks and undershirt to prevent skin irritation from straps; inspect skin under straps three times/day; massage under straps daily; feed with head elevated; use football hold when breastfeeding; hold and cuddle infant; provide appropriate toys and involve child in age-appropriate activities.

Developmental Dysplasia of Hip (DDH)

- **Signs/Symptoms:** Decreased abduction of affected leg; audible click when abducting or externally rotating affected hip; asymmetry of gluteal, popliteal, and thigh folds; apparent shortening of the femur; pelvis tilts downward on unaffected side when standing on affected extremity.
- **Treatment:** Brace; serial casts; surgical correction.
- **Nursing Interventions:**
  - Follow guidelines for clubfoot.
  - Infant with DDH: hip spica cast should be changed when needed (every 3–6 months).

Scoliosis

- **Signs/Symptoms:** Most often seen during preadolescent growth spurt via MD or school-based screening; scapular and hip heights are asymmetrical when child is viewed from behind; asymmetry and prominence of rib cage when bending forward; one breast may be larger; clothes do not fit well (uneven pants legs, crooked skirt hem).
- **Treatment:** Depends on extent, location, and type of curve; orthotics; spinal fusion for curves greater than 40 degrees; exercise to prevent atrophy of spinal and abdomen muscles.
- **Nursing Interventions:**
  - Teach purpose, function, application, and care of appliance.
  - Check skin for irritation.
  - Assist with clothing to disguise brace; encourage wearing brace for 16–23 hours per day for several years.
  - Encourage ventilation of feelings; role-play how to deal with reaction of others to brace.

Juvenile Idiopathic Arthritis

- **Signs/Symptoms:** Variable; one or more joints involved; joint swelling as a result of edema, joint effusion, and synovial thickening; stiffness in morning and after inactivity; loss of motion as a result of muscle spasms and joint inflammation; weakness and fatigue; spindle fingers with thick proximal joint and slender tip; joints may be painfree, tender, or painful; increased temperature; rash; uveitis; pericarditis; enlarged liver, spleen, lymph nodes.
- **Treatment:** Nonsteroidal inflammatory drugs (NSAIDs; no aspirin to prevent Reye's syndrome) to suppress inflammation; slower-acting

antirheumatic drugs; a biological agent that blocks cytokine tumor necrosis factor, interrupting inflammation; cytotoxic agents; corticosteroids used only when other medications are ineffective because of side effects; PT and OT to increase muscle strength, mobilize joints, prevent and correct deformities; splinting of knees, wrists, and hands to decrease pain and flexion deformities.

- **Nursing Interventions:**
  - Teach child to take medications as ordered, even during remissions.
  - Maintain functional alignment.
  - Apply heat as ordered.
  - Encourage independence in ADLs and exercise program; incorporate play in the program.
  - Balance activity/rest.
  - During exacerbations give medications to decrease pain; rest joints; maintain functional alignment; encourage isometric, not isotonic, exercises; maintain contact with school and peers; and support parents to cope with exacerbations, constant discomfort, risk of overindulgence, and seeking alternative therapies.

Geriatric Care

Geriatric Assessment Guidelines

- The most common physical ailments include:
  - Osteoarthritis
  - Hypertension
  - Heart disease
  - Hearing loss
  - Orthopedic impairments
  - Diabetes
- The leading causes of death for older adults are heart disease, cancer, and stroke.
- Be mindful that the elderly are not always hard of hearing.
- Speak to elderly clients in the same manner as any other adult client; do not speak to the elderly client as if he or she were a child.
- Eye contact instills confidence and will enable the client who is hearing impaired to better understand what is being said.

- Care should be taken to avoid unnecessary discomfort or injury during assessment.
- Be aware of generational differences; especially gender differences (i.e., modesty for females, independence for males).

Functional Assessment

- A comprehensive evaluation of the physical and cognitive abilities required to maintain independence.
- Assessment tools measure ADLs, instrumental ADLs, and psychological and social functioning.
- Comorbid conditions that negatively affect functional status include acute illness; alterations in nutrition and/or hydration; chronic illness; economics; environment; medications; psychiatric comorbidities; and psychological/social stressors.

Strategies to Promote/Maintain Optimal Function

- Schedule regular examinations for prevention and early detection of cancer, prevention of heart disease and stroke, and prevention and treatment of osteoarthritis.
- Optimize nutritional patterns.
- Maintain and enhance mental functioning.
- Enhance a sense of independence and productivity.
- Maintain and enhance social relationships and support.
- Maintain vaccination status.

Age-Related Changes	
↓ Skin thickness	More prone to skin breakdown; should be monitored more frequently for pressure ulcers.
↓ Skin vascularity	Altered thermoregulatory response increases risk of heat stroke.
↓ Subcutaneous tissue	Decreased insulation increases risk for hypothermia.
↓ Aortic elasticity	Increases diastolic blood pressure.
Calcification of thoracic wall	Obscured heart and lung sounds; displacement of apical pulse.

Continued

Age-Related Changes—*cont'd*	
↓ Nerve fibers/neurons	Allow extra time to comprehend, to learn, and to perform tasks.
↓ Nerve conduction	Response to pain is altered.
↓ Tactile sensation	Increases risk for self-injury.
↓ Hearing	Main causes: nerve deterioration, disease, environmental situations, medications, and cerumen impaction.
↓ Vision	Main causes: decreased pupil size and accommodation (alters visual accuracy), macular degeneration (impedes central vision), glaucoma (impedes peripheral vision), and cataracts (cloud vision).
↓ Speech	Main causes: stroke, dental difficulties, lack of teeth, and ill-fitting dentures.
↓ Touch/tactile stimulation	Main causes: fear, discomfort, stereotypes, sense of one's vulnerability, isolation.
↓ Movement	Main causes: osteoporosis, arthritis, lack of exercise, stroke, and weight gain.
↓ Taste/smell	Most older adults lose taste, especially for sweets, and the sense of smell; affects willingness to talk about food; reduces socialization of eating.
↓ Cognitive ability	Main causes: multidrug interactions and side effects of medications; forms of dementia (e.g., Alzheimer's disease); alcoholism; inadequate, broken sleep.

■ Assessing older adults for altered mental status is important. Use "3 D vision."
  ■ **Dementia:** cognitive deficits, such as lapse in memory, reasoning, and judgment.
  ■ **Delirium:** confusion/excitement marked by disorientation to time and place; usually accompanied by delusions and/or hallucinations.
  ■ **Depression:** diminished interest or pleasure in most or all activities; as many as 25% of nursing home residents are depressed.

Differentiating Delirium and Dementia

Factor	Delirium	Dementia
Onset	Sudden	Gradual
Duration	Brief (hours–day)	Long (months–years)
Causes	Infection, injury, intoxication, cerebrovascular accident, congestive heart failure, cerebral anoxia, medications, metabolic imbalances, myocardial infarction	Dehydration, depression, endocrine disorders, environmental change, electrolyte imbalance, medications, eye and ear problems, nutritional deficiencies, infection, fecal impaction, ischemia, insomnia, anemia
LOC	Fluctuates throughout day	Unaffected
Motor	Tremor, myoclonus, ataxia, hyperactivity	None until late
Speech	Incoherent	Normal to aphasic in later stage
Language	Vocabulary usual for client; frequent use of wrong words	Worsens as disorder progresses
Memory	Impaired	Impaired
Attention	Impaired, fluctuates	Normal to easily distracted
Perception	Hallucinations common	Hallucinations uncommon
Mood	Fearful, suspicious, irritable	Fearful, suspicious, irritable, depressed early in disorder
Sleep	Disturbances common	Disturbances common
General condition	Clients look sick	Clients look healthy
Clinical course	Fluctuates over short term	Stable over short term

Recommended Adult Immunization Schedule

Recommended Adult Immunization Schedule   UNITED STATES • 2009

Vaccine ▼ Age ▶	19–26 years	27–49 years	50–59 years	60–64 years	≥ 65 years
Diphtheria, Tetanus, Pertussis*	Substitute 1-time dose of Tdap for Td booster; then boost with Td every 10 yrs				Td booster every 10 yrs
Human Papillomavirus*	3 doses (females)				
Varicella*	2 doses				
Zoster				1 dose	
Measles, Mumps, Rubella*	1 or 2 doses		1 dose		
Influenza*			1 dose annually		
Pneumococcal	1 or 2 doses				1 dose
Hepatitis A*	2 doses				
Hepatitis B*	3 doses				
Meningococcal*	1 or more doses				

For all persons in this category who meet the age requirements and who lack evidence of immunity (e.g., lack documentation of vaccination or have no evidence of prior infection)

Recommended if some other risk factor is present (e.g., on the basis of medical, occupational, lifestyle, or other indications)

No recommendation

*Covered by the Vaccine Injury Compensation Program

Fall Risk Assessment and Prevention

Risk Factors	Prevention Strategies
Assessment data • Age >65 years • History of falls	• Monitor frequently. • Client should be close to nurses' station. • Implement facility fall prevention interventions.
Medications • Polypharmacy • CNS depressants • BP/HR-lowering meds • Diuretics and meds that ↑ intestinal motility	• Review medications with physician • Educate about use of sedative, hypnotic agents. • Suggest nonpharmacological treatment of symptoms if possible. • Assess medication interactions that may affect balance. • Instruct client/resident to avoid alcohol and sedatives. • Notify physician if medication makes client/resident ill or weak; inform physician about over-the-counter remedies, which can cause drowsiness and unsteadiness.
Mental status • Altered LOC • Disorientation	• Maintain a safe, structured environment. • Assess for subtle changes in stamina, social interaction, and ability to communicate, which could suggest a functional decline.
Cardiovascular • Postural hypotension	• Have client/resident rise slowly, perform ankle pumps or hand clenching, and raise head of bed before getting up. • Assess medications. • If necessary, have one person assist with standing.
Neurosensory • Visual impairment • Peripheral neuropathy • Difficulty with balance or gait	• Have yearly vision examinations. • Ensure proper footwear is worn. • Provide illumination at night. • Provide training in the use of assistive devices. • Provide balance training. • Refer to physical therapy if necessary.

Fall Risk Assessment and Prevention—*cont'd*

Risk Factors	Prevention Strategies
GI/GU • Incontinence • Urinary frequency • Diarrhea	• Ensure frequent toileting. • Mark pathway to bathroom. • Provide bedside commode.
Musculoskeletal • Decreased ROM • Amputee	• Provide strength and balance training. • Provide range-of-motion exercises. • Provide appropriate assistive devices.
Assistive devices • Canes • Walkers • Wheelchairs	• Ensure that such devices are not damaged and are appropriately sized. • Teach client/resident to use appropriate assistive devices correctly and at all times.
Environment • Cluttered room • Tubes and lines	• Minimize clutter and remove unnecessary equipment. • Ensure call light is within easy reach.

Nursing Interventions

■ Do not move client/resident if he or she is unconscious, complains of severe pain, or has a deformity of an extremity (obvious fracture, internal rotation of hip or knee).

■ Assess LOC and orientation, ability to move all extremities, VS, pain level, alignment and symmetry of extremities, and soft tissue and skin (check for abrasions, swelling, or deformity).

■ Assist client/resident to bed or chair if there are no obvious injuries and client/resident is alert and able to communicate; get assistance.

■ Call physician or nursing supervisor.

■ Treat minor injuries:
  ■ Clean and dress abrasions.
  ■ Apply ice to contusions or areas of swelling.

■ Assess for acute underlying condition, such as infection, transient ischemic attack, urinary tract infection, hypotension, and cardiac dysrhythmia.

■ Assess for orthostasis, problems with gait, changes in mental status, and recent changes in functional status.

- Review records for preexisting conditions, medication use, and previous falls.
- Assess location of fall for environmental hazards.
- Document:
  - How you found the client/resident
  - The client's condition, including mental status, vital signs, complaints of pain, comments about what caused fall, and observable injuries
  - Interventions provided
  - Who was notified and responses by supervisors or physician
  - Follow-up assessments
- Monitor client/resident closely for changes in condition, especially changes in mental status, which can suggest brain injury.

Preventing Falls in the Home

Floors
- Move the furniture so natural walkways are clear.
- Remove throw rugs, or use double-sided tape or a nonslip backing so rugs do not slip.
- Keep objects off the floor.
- Coil or tape cords and wires next to wall.

Stairs and Steps
- Keep objects off stairs; fix loose or uneven steps.
- Install overhead light at the top and bottom of stairs.
- Install a light switch at the top and bottom of stairs.
- Fix loose handrails; install handrails running the length of the stairs on both sides of stairway.
- Make sure carpet is firmly attached at each stair step.
- Remove loose carpet, and attach nonslip rubber treads on stairs.

Kitchen
- Keep often-used items on lower shelves (about waist high).
- Keep a steady step stool with a grip bar available.

Bedroom/Bath
- Place a lamp close to the bed where it is easy to reach.
- Light entire path from bed to bathroom.

- Put a nonslip rubber mat or self-stick strips on floor of tub or shower.
- Install grab bar inside tub and next to toilet.

Medications and the Elderly

Age-Related Changes in Medication Effects

Function	Physiological Change	Changes in Effect
Absorption	↓ Intestinal motility; ↓ blood flow to the gut	Delayed peak effect Delayed signs and symptoms of toxicity
Distribution	↓ Body water; ↑ percentage of body fat; ↓ amount of plasma proteins; ↓ lean body mass	↑ Serum concentration of water-soluble drugs; ↑ half-life of fat-soluble drugs; ↑ amount of active drug; ↑ drug concentration
Metabolism	↓ Blood flow to liver; ↓ liver function	↓ Rate of drug clearance by the liver; ↑ accumulation of some drugs
Excretion	↓ Kidney function; ↓ creatinine clearance	↑ Accumulation of drugs that are normally excreted by the liver

Polypharmacy
- Polypharmacy is the concurrent use of several medications.
- Taking two medications increases the risk of an adverse drug event by 6%.
- Taking eight medications increases the risk of an adverse drug event by 100%.

Causes
- Taking unnecessary medications.
- Duplication: Taking different medications for the same reason.
- Concurrent use of interacting medications.
- Taking contraindicated medications.
- Taking medications to treat the side effects of other medications.
- Medications are not discontinued after problem has resolved.

- Take a complete medication history including OTC drugs; herbal and natural supplements.
- Encourage the use of one pharmacy for all prescriptions.
- Have pharmacy and physician review medications regularly.
- Help client to develop a simple medication regimen.
- Coordinate care if client sees more than one physician.
- Encourage nonpharmacological treatments whenever possible.

Communicating With Impaired Geriatric Clients

Hearing Impairment
- Get older adult's attention.
- If he or she is wearing a hearing aid, check the volume setting.
- If the older adult is not wearing a hearing aid, check to see if he or she can hear better out of one ear than the other. If so, speak to that side.
- Ask whether the older adult can read lips or can communicate in sign language.
- Speak up but do not shout; use lower-pitched tones because they are heard more easily than higher ones.
- Speak slowly and clearly and emphasize key words; keep your mouth in clear view, and maintain eye contact.
- Use other channels of communication (e.g., gestures, diagrams) and printed materials and writing implements (e.g., chalkboards and paper and pencil).
- Alert the older adult when you are changing the subject.

Visual Impairment
- Identify yourself clearly.
- Inform the older adult when you are entering or leaving the room.
- Use clear language when you give directions.
- Obtain and encourage the use of low-vision aids.
- If an older adult wears glasses, make sure they are available.
- When using print material, make sure that it is a size the older adult can read.

Speech Impairment

- Show the older adult immediately that you do not expect him or her to speak well, but encourage them to do the best they can.
- Provide alternate forms of communication.
- Encourage the older adult to use gestures and body language.

Movement and Tactile Impairment

- Be aware of movement limitations.
- Be aware of pain and its impact on the older adult's range of movement.
- Gestures are effective communication tools, particularly with the hard of hearing.
- Touch is reassuring and should be used if acceptable to client and caregiver.

Cognitive Impairment

- Keep interaction simple; use one-step commands.
- Use closed, not open-ended, questions.
- Use simple sentences.
- Don't ask questions that rely on good memory.

Age-Related Conditions

Alzheimer's Disease

Alzheimer's disease (AD) is the most common cause of elderly dementia and represents half of all dementias. It is a disabling degenerative disease of the nervous system with a disease process that starts long before symptoms appear. Early-onset AD may begin as early as 40 years of age; late-onset AD begins after age 60. It is characterized by dementia and failure of memory for recent events and results in total incapacitation and death. Life expectancy after development of symptoms is 8–10 years

- **Causes:** Unknown.
- **Signs/Symptoms:**
  - *Stage I:* loss of recent memory; easily irritated; loss of interest in life; decline of abstract thinking and problem-solving abilities.
  - *Stage II:* most common stage when diagnosed; profound memory deficits; inability to concentrate or manage business or personal affairs.

- **Stage III:** aphasia; inability to recognize or use objects; involuntary emotional outbursts; incontinence.
- **Stage IV:** nonverbal and withdrawn; loss of appetite leading to state of emaciation; all body functions cease; death ensues.

■ **Treatment:** No cure; four drugs are FDA-approved to treat AD by helping to maintain thinking, memory, and speaking skills.
  ■ *Mild to moderate AD:* donepezil (Aricept®); rivastigmine (Excelon®); galantamine (Razadyne®).
  ■ *Moderate to severe AD:* donepezil (Aricept®); memantine (Namenda®).

■ **Nursing Interventions:**
  ■ Monitor VS and LOC; implement collaborative care as ordered.
  ■ Keep requests simple and avoid confrontation.
  ■ Maintain a consistent environment and frequently reorient client.
  ■ Provide client and family with literature on AD.
  ■ Advise family that, as AD progresses, so does the need for supervision.
  ■ Recommend that client wear bracelet in case he or she becomes lost.
  ■ Advise family to secure windows and doors to prevent wandering.
  ■ Explain actions, dosages, side effects, and adverse reactions of medications.

Dehydration in Older Adults

■ **Causes:** When the amount of water leaving the body exceeds the amount of water taken in by the body.

■ **Risk factors:** >85 years of age; nursing home resident; difficulty with feeding/swallowing; dementia; multiple chronic conditions; multiple medications; vomiting or diarrhea; confined to bed; diuretic or laxative use; self-restriction of fluids related to incontinence or nighttime voiding.

■ **Signs/Symptoms:**
  ■ Confusion and change in level of consciousness.
  ■ Tachycardia, orthostatic hypotension, and elevated temperature.
  ■ Low urine output and dark-yellow to brownish urine.
  ■ Dry skin, poor skin turgor, and dry mucous membrane.
  ■ Constipation, fecal impaction.
  ■ Dizziness.
  ■ Infection.

- Weakness, fatigue.
- Signs of electrolyte imbalance.
- Poor skin turgor over forehead or sternum (do not use hand or arm because it is unreliable).
- Increased urinary specific gravity.
- Increased hematocrit.

- **Treatment:** PO and NG fluids; hypotonic and isotonic IV fluids.
- **Nursing Interventions:**
  - Evaluate hydration status by assessing VS, urine specific gravity; BUN; CBC; I&O.
  - Offer a variety of fluids and have client/resident take sips throughout the day if he or she has trouble taking more at a time.
  - Document I&O and difficulties drinking.
  - Assess and record weight daily.
  - Post the volume of each container (e.g., cups, bowls, and tea cups) in the client/resident's room.
  - If client/resident requires test preparation (NPO or bowel cleansing), arrange timing so that test occurs as soon as possible. Offer fluids immediately after test is completed unless contraindicated. Consider IV hydration if NPO status is prolonged.
  - Notify physician immediately if signs and symptoms of dehydration are present. Dehydration can progress quickly and become severe and is associated with a high mortality rate in older adult clients/residents.

Malnutrition in Older Adults

- **Causes:** Inadequate intake of protein, carbohydrates, nutrients, and/or minerals.
- **Risk Factors:** Eating less than one half the meals or snacks served; complaints of mouth pain; dentures do not fit; difficulty chewing or swallowing; trouble with using utensils; is confused, wanders, or paces; needs help to eat or drink; has diabetes, pulmonary disease, cancer, or other chronic disease; has limited income for food and medicine; depression; medications that decrease appetite, cause constipation, or cause drowsiness during meal time.
- **Signs/Symptoms:**
  - Swollen or inflamed eyelids.
  - Angular wrinkles emerging out of the mouth.

- Sores and reddening inside mouth; disappearance of taste buds.
- Swollen thyroid gland.
- Emaciation and muscular atrophy.
- Dull, yellow appearance to skin; xerosis.
- Swelling of gums; tooth decay.
- Unresponsive and disinterested in surroundings; irritable; poor memory.
- **Nursing Interventions:**
  - Provide oral care before meals (make sure mouth is clean and teeth fit properly).
  - Encourage eating six small meals each day.
  - Offer many kinds of foods and beverages.
  - Provide assistance to those who have trouble feeding themselves.
  - Allow sufficient time to finish eating.
  - Keep ongoing record of resident's/client's weight.
  - Review appropriate labs.
  - Consider consultation with dietitian, dentist, physician, or occupational therapist or social worker.
  - Reassess dietary restrictions.
  - Recommend higher-calorie food, beverages, or oral supplements.
  - Give high-calorie liquids with medications.
  - Incorporate more fluid into diet plan unless restricted because of kidney problems.

Pressure Ulcers

- **Causes:** Breakdown of skin resulting from staying in one position too long without a shift in body weight.
- **Risk Factors:** Degenerative neurologic/neuromuscular disease; cerebrovascular disease; brain or spinal cord injury; depression; drugs that adversely affect alertness; pain; use of restraints; protein-calorie undernutrition; edema; diabetes mellitus; peripheral vascular disease; COPD; bowel and bladder incontinence.
- **Signs/Symptoms:**
  - *Stage I:* reddened area on the skin that, when pressed, is "non-blanchable" (does not turn white); indicates that a pressure ulcer is starting to develop.
  - *Stage II:* skin blisters or forms an open sore; area around the sore may be red and irritated.

- **_Stage III:_** skin breakdown now looks like a crater; there is damage to the tissue below the skin.
- **_Stage IV:_** pressure ulcer has become so deep that there is damage to the muscle, bone, tendons, and/or joints.
- **Treatment:** Debridement; wound cleansing; irrigation; dressings; adjuvant therapies.
- **Prevention:**
  - Inspect skin daily and document findings.
  - Effectively manage urinary and fecal incontinence.
  - Clean skin promptly using a mild, nonirritating, nondrying cleansing solution. Avoid friction during cleansing.
  - Use topical moisture barriers and moisture-absorbing pad for clients who are incontinent.
  - Position client to alleviate pressure and shearing forces.
  - Reposition client every 2 hours when in bed and every hour when in a chair.
  - Teach client to shift his or her weight every 15 minutes while in a chair.
  - Use positioning devices and foam padding. Do not use donut-shaped devices.
  - Avoid placing the client on his or her trochanters or directly on a wound.
  - Maintain the lowest head elevation possible to prevent sacral pressure.
  - Use lifting devices, such as draw sheets or a trapeze.
  - Prevent contractures. Provide adequate nutrition and hydration.
  - Do not massage reddened areas over bony prominence.
- **Nursing Interventions:**
  - Follow facility's policies or protocols for dressing changes.
  - Clean the wound with each dressing change. Use normal saline to clean ulcers. Avoid using skin cleansers and antiseptic solutions.
  - Follow infection control techniques. Use clean gloves.
  - **Wash hands before and after wound care.**
  - Use effective pain control measures, including additional dosing for debridement or dressing changes, if indicated.
  - Recommend modified food texture or temperature to increase intake.
  - Assess side effects of medications that may decrease appetite.

- Administer medications that cause drowsiness after mealtimes, if possible.
- Treat side effects if medications cannot be changed.
- Document and report assessments, interventions, and outcomes.

End of Life

End-of-Life Choices
- The client and/or family members will need to decide if the client chooses to have cardiopulmonary resuscitation (CPR) or a Do Not Resuscitate (DNR) order.
- In the final weeks of life, actively dying clients and/or family members will need to decide if artificial feeding and artificial hydration can be started.
- The client and/or family members will need to decide if the client shall remain at home during the dying process or enter the hospital until death occurs.

Changes Expected in the Dying Process
- The closer to death, the client has a decreased desire to eat.
- Dyspnea occurs toward the end of life.
- Saliva collected at the back of the throat is called the "death rattle."
- As death approaches, some experience a high fever; others feel cold; feet and legs may become cyanotic and mottled. This is an indicator that death will occur in a few hours.
- Urine output will decrease, become dark in color, and have a strong odor.

Nursing Interventions
- Monitor respiratory rate.
- Administer diuretics or antibodies as ordered.
- Explain to the family members the changes expected in the dying process.
- Plan activities to conserve energy.
- Place client upright in the bed or in a recliner with pillows to 45 degrees.
- Offer alternative comfort measures, such as a massage and muscle relaxation.
- Administer oxygen if ordered.

- Place a fan in the client's room if requested by the client.
- Administer low-dose morphine as ordered.
- Place a humidifier in the room. If secretions are copious, suction client as needed.
- Allow the client to choose when and what to eat.
- Provide frequent mouth care with sponge-tipped toothettes.
- Apply lanolin to dry, cracked lips.
- Assess for agitation, pain, or other discomfort.
- If the cause of the agitation cannot be determined, try medication for pain.
- Keep the client safe by keeping side rails up.
- Keep perineal area clean and dry by checking the pad or the diaper frequently.
- Assure family members that the client may become confused.
- When providing care, always speak to the client as if he or she can hear. Hearing is the last sense that one loses.
- Provide a quiet environment where each loved one can say goodbye in a way that will reflect their culture and values.
- Allow time for prayers and ceremonies based on the client and family's culture and values.

Mental Health

Mental health is defined as a state of successful performance of mental function, resulting in productive activities, fulfilling relationships with other people, and the ability to adapt to change and cope with adversity.

Personality Development

	Erikson's Developmental Stages		
Stage	**Age**	**Positive Outcomes**	**Negative Outcomes**
Trust vs. Mistrust	Birth to 18 months	Strong bonds; trust in mothering figure	Inability to bond; insecure; distrustful
Autonomy vs. Shame or Doubt	18 months to 3 years	Independence; some self-esteem	Doubtful of own ability; dependent
Initiative vs. Guilt	3 to 6 years	Sense of purpose and ability	Immobilized by guilt; dependent
Industry vs. Inferiority	6 to 12 years	Self-confidence by doing and achieving	Sense of inferiority; inability to achieve
Identity vs. Role Confusion	12 to 20 years	Secure sense of self; positive ideals	Confusion; inability to make decisions
Intimacy vs. Isolation	20 to 30 years	Lasting relationship or commitment	Isolation and fear of commitment
Generativity vs. Stagnation	30 to 65 years	Creates a family; considers future welfare of others	Stagnation; self-centered; unfulfilled life and career
Ego Integrity vs. Despair	65 years to death	Positive sense of self-worth; accepts and prepares for death	Feeling of hopelessness; fears and denies death

251

Freud's Stages of Personality Development

Stage	Age	Positive Outcomes	Negative Outcomes
Oral Stage	Birth to 18 months	• Focus of energy is the mouth. • Fulfillment of basic needs. • Sense of security and ability to trust others.	• Mother's anxiety may be passed on to infant. • Insecure and unable to trust.
Anal Stage	18 months to 3 years	• Focus is on excretory functions. • Learns independence and control. • Permissive, accepting toilet training results in feelings of importance. • Child becomes extroverted, productive, altruistic.	• Strict and rigid toilet training may produce traits such as stubbornness, stinginess, and miserliness. • Allowing defecation at inappropriate times or in an inappropriate manner may produce traits such as cruelty, destructiveness, or untidiness.
Phallic Stage	3 to 6 years	• Focus of energy is on genitalia. • Characterized by child's unconscious desire to eliminate same-sex parent. • Internal conflict resolves with development of strong identification with same-sex parent.	• Feelings of guilt. • Failure to identify with same-sex parent. • Failure to adopt attitudes, beliefs, and value systems of same-sex parent. • Egocentric.

Continued

Freud's Stages of Personality Development—*cont'd*

Stage	Age	Positive Outcomes	Negative Outcomes
Latency Stage	6 to 12 years	• Energy focus changes from egocentric to socialization with peers. • Healthy same-sex relationships.	• Remains egocentric. • Difficulty being accepted by peer group. • Self-gratification.
Genital Stage	13 to 20 years	• Focus of energy is on relationships with opposite sex. • Prepares to select a mate. • Adopts behaviors acceptable by societal norms.	• Self-serving. • Unable to form healthy relationships with opposite sex.

Psychological Assessment

- **Safety:** Your safety ALWAYS comes first.
- **Exit:** Always position yourself between the client and an exit. Never allow a client to block your means of escape.
- **Awareness:** Observe for nonverbal signs of aggression or violence, such as clenched fists, profanity, pacing, raised tone of voice, ↑ respiratory rate, wide-eyed stare, verbal threats, and/or weapons.
- **Be assertive:** Make your boundaries known; set limits; be consistent; avoid bargaining or arguing with clients.

Mental Status Assessment

Component	Documentation
Affect	External expression of emotional state: friendly; hostile; euphoric; sad; despondent. Should be congruent with mood; may be incongruent with psychiatric disorders.
Appearance	Grooming; hygiene; posture; eye contact; correlation between appearance and developmental stage/age.
General Attitude	Cooperative; uncooperative; friendly; hostile; defensive; guarded; apathetic.
Impulse Control	Aggression; fear; guilt; affection; sexual.
Judgment/Insight	Decision-making and problem-solving ability; coping.
Mood	Depressed; sad; anxious; fearful; labile; irritable; elated; euphoric; guilty; despair.
Motor Activity	Tremors; tics; mannerisms; gestures; gait; hyperactivity; restlessness; agitation; rigid.
Perceptual Disturbances	Hallucinations (auditory, visual, tactile, olfactory, gustatory); illusions.
Speech Pattern	Aphasia; volume; impairments; stutter.
Sensory/Cognitive	Alertness; orientation; memory; abstract thinking.
Thought Process	**Form of thought:** attention span; "word salads;" echolalia. **Content of thought:** delusional; suicidal; homicidal; obsessive; paranoid; suspicious; phobic.

Grief

- Intense emotional anguish in response to a perceived, significant personal loss.
- Brief response is a period of *mourning*; the normal mourning process is adaptive and characterized by feelings of sadness, guilt, anger, helplessness, hopelessness, and despair; lasts from weeks to years.

Kübler-Ross's Stages of Grief

Stage	Responses	Nursing Implications
Denial	"Not me!" Unable to believe loss.	• Explore own feelings about death. • Encourage communication.
Anger	"Why me?" Resists loss with hostility and anger.	• Recognize anger as a form of coping. • Do not abandon or become defensive.
Bargaining	"Yes, me, but..." Barters for time; expresses guilt for past behaviors.	• Assist with ventilation of feelings. • Help resolve unfinished business, if appropriate.
Depression	"Yes, me." Realizes full impact of loss; may talk, withdraw, cry, or feel lonely.	• Convey caring. • Acknowledge sad feelings. • Accept and support grieving.
Acceptance	"OK, me." Accepts loss; may have ↓ interest in activities and people; may be peaceful and quiet.	• Help family understand and allow client's withdrawal. • Support family's participation in care. • Do not abandon client and family.

Maladaptive Grief Responses

■ *Prolonged response:* Characterized by an intense preoccupation with memories of the lost entity for many years after the loss has occurred.

■ *Delayed response:* Individual becomes fixed in the denial stage of the grieving process; may develop anxiety, eating, and/or sleeping disorders.

■ *Distorted response:* Individual becomes fixed in the anger stage of the grieving process; consumed with overwhelming despair; unable to perform ADLs; may develop pathological depression.

Information Disclosure
- Clients have the right to receive accurate, easily understood information and assistance in making informed health-care decisions about their health plans, professionals, and facilities.

Choice of Providers/Plans
- Clients have the right to a choice of health-care providers that is sufficient to ensure access to appropriate high-quality health care.

Access to Emergency Services
- Clients have the right to access emergency health-care services when and where the need arises.
- Health plans should provide payment when a client presents to an emergency department with acute symptoms of sufficient severity that a "prudent layperson" could reasonably expect the absence of medical attention to result in serious jeopardy, serious impairment to bodily functions, or serious dysfunction of any bodily organ or part.

Participation in Treatment Decisions
- Clients have the right and responsibility to fully participate in all decisions related to their health care.
- Clients who are unable to fully participate in treatment decisions have the right to be represented by parents, guardians, family members, or other conservators.
- Clients have the right to accept or refuse treatment to the extent permitted by the law and to be informed of the medical consequences of their actions. In some emergency situations, clients can be medicated or treated against their will, but state laws vary.

Respect and Nondiscrimination
- Clients have the right to considerate, respectful care from all members of the health-care system at all times and under all circumstances.
- An environment of mutual respect is essential to maintain a quality health-care system.

- Clients have the right to communicate with health-care providers in confidence and to have the confidentiality of their individually identifiable health-care information protected.
- Clients have the right to review and copy their own medical records and request amendments to their records.

Complaints and Appeals

- All consumers have the right to a fair and efficient process for resolving differences with their health plans, health-care providers, and the institutions that serve them.

Client Responsibilities

- In a health-care system that protects client rights, it is reasonable to expect and encourage clients to assume reasonable responsibilities.
  - Greater individual involvement by clients in their care increases the likelihood of achieving the best outcomes and helps support a quality improvement, cost-conscious environment.

Commitment to a Psychiatric Facility

Types of Commitment

Voluntary

An individual decides he or she needs treatment and admits himself or herself to a treatment facility and leaves of own volition—unless a professional (psychiatrist/other professional) decides that the person is a danger to self or to others.

Involuntary

- Emergency:
  - Involves imminent danger to self or others; person has demonstrated a clear and present danger to self or others.
  - Usually initiated by health professionals, authorities, and sometimes friends or family; requires assessment by two mental health professionals.
  - Person is threatening to harm self or others, or evidence exists that the person is unable to care for herself or himself (nourishment, personal, medical, safety), with reasonable probability that death will result within a month.

- Civil or judicial commitment:
    - Longer than emergency commitment.
    - To provide treatment to clients or to protect public.
    - Procedures vary according to state laws.

Confidentiality

Confidentiality Issues

- Confidentiality is important in all areas of health care, but notably so in psychiatry because of possible discriminatory treatment of those with mental illness. All individuals have a right to privacy, and all client records and communications should be kept confidential.
- Clients are protected by the Health Insurance Portability and Accountability Act (HIPAA).
- Do not discuss clients by using their actual names or client-specific identifiers.
- Be sensitive to the rights of the clients and their right to confidentiality.
- Do not discuss client particulars outside of a private, professional environment; do not discuss with family members or friends.
- Be particularly careful during conversations in elevators of hospitals or community centers. You never know who might be on the elevator with you.
- Even in educational presentations, protect the client's identity by changing names and obtaining all permissions (e.g., informed consents).
- Every client has the right to confidential and respectful treatment.
- Accurate, objective record-keeping is important; documentation is legally significant when implementing client care.
- If not documented, treatments have legally not been performed.

When Confidentiality Must Be Breached

- **Child abuse:**
    - If suspected or clear that a child is being abused or in danger of abuse (physical/sexual/emotional) or neglect, the health professional must report such abuse as mandated by the Child Abuse Prevention Treatment Act (PL-93-247), originally enacted in 1974.
- **Elder abuse:**
    - If suspected or clear that an elder is being abused or in danger of abuse or neglect, then the health professional must report this abuse.

■ **Tarasoff principle:**

■ This principle refers to the responsibility of a therapist, health professional, or nurse to warn a potential victim of imminent danger (a threat to harm person) and breach confidentiality.

■ The person in danger and others (able to protect person) must be notified of the intended harm.

Restraints and Seclusion

■ The Joint Commission advocates reducing the use of behavioral restraints and has set forth guidelines for safety when restraints are used.

■ In an emergency situation, restraints may be applied by an authorized and qualified nonlicensed independent practitioner (UAP) staff member.

■ Once a restraint has been applied, the following timeframes must be used for reevaluation/reordering:

■ Within the first hour after application of restraint, a physician or licensed practitioner (LP) must evaluate the client.

■ After the first 4-hour order expires, a qualified RN or other authorized staff person must reevaluate the individual and the need to continue restraint/seclusion must be established.

■ If restraint/seclusion is still needed, a licensed practitioner must be notified and an order (written/verbal) must be given for 4 additional hours of restraint/seclusion.

■ After 8 hours of restraint/seclusion, a face-to-face evaluation of continued need must be completed by a licensed practitioner. If needed, another 4 hours may be ordered (written).

■ Evaluations may be repeated as long as restraint and seclusion are clinically necessary.

Alert: Restraint of a client, which may be physical or chemical, infringes on a client's freedom of movement and may result in injury (physical or psychological) or death.

Abuse

Child Abuse

Signs of Child Abuse

Physical Abuse	Sexual Abuse
• Pattern of bruises/welts. • Burns (e.g., from cigarettes, scalds). • Lesions resembling bites or fingernail marks. • Unexplained fractures or dislocations, especially in child younger than 3 years old. • Areas of baldness from hair pulling. • Injuries in various stages of healing. • Other injuries or untreated illness, unrelated to present injury. • X-rays revealing old fractures.	• Signs of genital irritation, such as pain or itching. • Bruised or bleeding genitalia. • Enlarged vaginal or rectal orifice. • Stains and/or blood on underwear. • Unusual sexual behavior.

Signs Common to Both Physical and Sexual Child Abuse

• Signs of "failure to thrive" syndrome. • Details of injury changing from person to person. • History inconsistent with developmental stages. • Parent blaming child or sibling for injury. • Parental anger toward child for injury. • Parental hostility toward health-care workers	• Exaggeration or absence of emotional response from parent regarding child's injury. • Parent not providing child with comfort. • Toddler or preschooler not protesting parent's leaving. • Child showing preference for health-care worker over parent.

Child Abuser Characteristics

- Stressful living situation (e.g., unemployment).
- Poor coping strategies; suspiciousness or tendency to lose temper easily.
- Isolated; few or no support systems.
- Lack of understanding of the needs of children (e.g., basic care, child development).
- Expectation of perfection from child; tendency to blow child's behavior out of proportion.

Child Incest

Incest often involves a father–daughter relationship (biological/stepfather), but it can also involve a father–son or mother–son relationship.

Behavioral Patterns of Incest Abusers

- Attempts to make child feel special ("it is our special secret"); gift giving.
- Favoritism (becoming intimate friend/sex partner; replacing mother/other parent).
- Serious boundary violations and no safe place for the child (child's bedroom usually used).
- Threats to prevent child from telling about the sexual activities.

Signs of Incest

- Low self-esteem, sexual acting out, mood changes, and sudden poor performance in school on the part of the child.
- Parent spending inordinate amount of time with child, especially in room or late at night, and being very attentive to child.
- Apprehensiveness in the child (fearing sexual act/retaliation).
- Possible use of alcohol and drugs.

All child abuse or child neglect must be reported.

Domestic Violence/Partner Abuse

Cycle of Battering
Phase I (Tension Building)
- Anger expressed with little provocation; minor battering occurs and excuses are made.
- Tension mounts and victim tries to placate batterer.
- Victim assumes guilt.

Phase II (Acute Battering)
- Period is most violent; may last up to 24 hours.
- Beating may be severe, and victim may provoke batterer to get it over with.
- Battering minimized by abuser.
- Help sought by victim if abuse is life threatening or safety of children is threatened.

Phase III (Calm, Loving, Respite)
- Batterer is loving, kind, and contrite.
- Batterer becomes fearful of victim leaving.
- Lesson has been taught, and now batterer believes victim "understands."
- Victim believes batterer can change, and batterer uses guilt. Victim believes this (calm/loving in phase III) is what batterer is really like. Victim hopes the previous phases will not repeat themselves.
- Victim stays because of fear for life (batterer threatens more and self-esteem is reduced), society valuing marriage, divorce being viewed negatively, and financial dependence.

This cycle then starts all over again, resulting in a dangerous situation in which the victim often is killed.

Domestic Abuse Safety/Escape Plan
- Rehearse exit plan (doors, windows, elevators).
- Have a place to go to be and feel safe (friends, relatives, motel).
- Pack a survival kit that includes:
  - Money (cab)
  - Change of clothes
  - Identifying information (passports, birth certificate)
  - Legal documents, including protection orders
  - Address books
  - Jewelry
  - Important papers
- Start an individual checking or savings account.
- Always have a safe exit; do not argue in areas with no exit.
  - Know how to contact domestic abuse/legal hotlines to protect victim's legal rights.
  - Review safety/escape plan consistently (monthly).

Elder Abuse

Types of Elder Abuse
- Elder neglect (lack of care by omission or commission).
- Psychological or emotional abuse (verbal assaults, insults, threats).
- Physical abuse (physical injury, infliction of pain, use of drugs and restraints).
- Sexual abuse (nonconsensual sex, rape, sodomy).
- Financial abuse (misuse of resources: social security, property).
- Self-neglect (elder cannot provide appropriate self-care).

Physical Signs
- Hematomas, welts, bites, burns, bruises, and pressure sores.
- Fractures (various stages of healing), contractures.
- Rashes, fecal impaction.
- Weight loss, dehydration, substandard personal hygiene.
- Broken dentures, hearing aids, and other devices; poor oral hygiene; traumatic alopecia; subconjunctival hemorrhage.

Caregiver Behavioral Signs
- Insistence on being present during entire appointment.
- Answering for client.
- Expressing indifference or anger; not offering assistance.
- Not visiting hospitalized client.

Abused Elder Characteristics
- Hesitation to be open; appearing fearful; poor eye contact; shame; baby talk.
- Paranoia, anxiety, anger, low self-esteem.
- Contractures, inconsistent medication regimen (subtherapeutic levels), malnutrition, poor hygiene, dehydration.
- Signing over power of attorney (unwillingly); possessions gone; lack of money.

Other Kinds of Abuse

Emotional Neglect
Behaviors of an emotionally neglectful parent/caretaker include:
- Ignoring the child.
- Ignoring the child's needs (social, educational, and developmental).

- Rebuffing the child's attempts at establishing interactions that are meaningful.
- Providing little to no positive reinforcement.

Emotional Injury

Emotional injury results in serious impairment to the child's functioning on all levels. It may include the following characteristics:

- Caregiver treatment of the child that is harsh; cruel and negative comments; belittling of the child.
- Behavior that is immature or inappropriate for the child's age.
- Anxiety, fearfulness, and sleep disturbances.
- Inappropriate affect, self-destructive behaviors.
- Possible isolating behavior, stealing, and cheating (as indication of emotional injury).

Male Sexual Abuse

Males can be sexually abused by mothers, fathers, uncles, pedophiles, and others in authority (e.g., coach, teacher, minister, priest).

Problems experienced by male victims of sexual abuse include:

- Depression, shame, blame, guilt, and other emotional effects of child sexual abuse.
- Issues related to masculinity, isolation, and struggles with seeking or receiving help.

Psychiatric Disorders

Anxiety Disorders

Four Levels of Anxiety

1. **Mild:** Can positively motivate someone to perform at a high level by helping him or her to focus on the situation at hand.
2. **Moderate:** Reduces the perceptual field; creates trouble in attending to the person's surroundings, although he or she can follow commands/directions.
3. **Severe:** Results in an inability to attend to his or her surroundings; leads to possible development of physical symptoms, such as sweating and palpitations.
4. **Panic:** A state of terror in which the only concern is escape; communication impossible at this point.

Types of Anxiety Disorders

Generalized Anxiety Disorder

- Excessive anxiety for 6 months or more.
- Hypervigilance; difficult to control worry.
- Three or more of the following symptoms:
  - Restlessness; irritability
  - Easily fatigued
  - ↓ Concentration
  - ↑ Muscle tension
  - Tachycardia; chest tightness
  - Sleep disturbance
  - Tremors
  - Dizziness
  - Diaphoresis

Panic Disorder

- Panic attacks lasting from 10 minutes to 30 minutes.
- Distorted perception.
- Erratic behavior; combative; withdrawn.
- Incoherent communication.
- Panic stricken, angry, terrified mood.
- Dyspnea, pallor, hypotension.

Agoraphobia

- Unrealistic fear of open spaces.

Social Phobia

- Unrealistic fear of social gatherings/events/groups of people.

Obsessive-Compulsive Disorder

- Characterized by intrusive, repetitive thoughts.
- Results in compulsive behaviors that the person feels compelled to perform to alleviate anxiety.

Posttraumatic Stress Disorder

- A severe and ongoing emotional reaction to an extreme psychological trauma.
- Characterized by flashbacks, nightmares, and avoidance of stimuli associated with the traumatic event.

Client/Family Education

- Educate client and family members about the stages of anxiety.
- Stress the importance of early diagnosis and treatment because these are chronic illnesses that become worse and more difficult to treat over time.
- Explain to the client and family the need for ongoing management.
- Many of these disorders are frustrating to family members. Family therapy may be needed to negotiate and agree on living arrangements that respect the needs of the client and all family members.
- As in all chronic disorders, remissions and exacerbations will be experienced.
- Reinforce with families that they also need support and sometimes a respite from the situation.

Eating Disorders

- Influenced by many factors, including family rituals and values around food and eating, ethnic and cultural influences, societal influences, and individual biology.
- American society currently stresses physical beauty and fitness and favors the thin and slim female as the ideal.
- There has been a dramatic increase in the number of people who are obese in the United States; the rate of increase among children has been especially alarming.

Anorexia Nervosa

- Clients are obsessed with losing weight and believe that they are overweight, even though they are emaciated.
- Symptoms include:
  - Body weight 85% or less than ideal body weight for height, build, and age
  - An intense and overwhelming fear of gaining weight or becoming fat
  - Body mass index of 18.5 or less
  - Amenorrhea develops, as defined by the absence of three consecutive menstrual cycles

Bulimia Nervosa

- Clients use/manipulate eating behaviors in an effort to control weight.
- Symptoms include:
  - Recurrent binge eating of a large amount of food over a short time period
  - Lack of control
  - Self-induced vomiting, laxative use, fasting, and exercise
  - Normal weight (some underweight/overweight)
  - Tooth enamel erosion; finger or pharynx bruising

Client/Family Education

- Client and family need to understand the serious nature of both disorders.
  - Mortality rate for anorexia nervosa is 2%-8%.
  - About 50% of those with bulimia nervosa recover with treatment.
- A team approach is important. The team should or may include a nutritionist, psychiatrist, therapist, physician, psychiatric nurse, eating disorder specialist, and others.
- Client and family need to be involved with the team.
- Teach client coping strategies, allow for expression of feelings, teach relaxation techniques, and help with ways (other than food) to feel in control.
- Family therapy is important to work out parent–child issues, especially concerning control.
- Focus on the fact that clients do recover and improve, and encourage patience when there is a behavioral setback.

Mood Disorders

Related to a person's emotional tone or affective state, can have an effect on behavior and influence a person's personality and world view in the following ways:

- Extremes of mood (mania or depression) can have devastating consequences on the client, family, and society.
- These consequences include financial, legal, marital, relationship, employment, spiritual losses and despair that results in potential suicide and death.

Depressive Disorders
Major Depressive Disorder (Unipolar Depression)
- Involves at least 2 weeks of depression/loss of interest and four additional depressive symptoms, with one or more major depressive episodes.

Dysthymic Disorder
- An ongoing, low-grade depression of at least 2 years' duration for more days than not that does not meet the criteria for major depression.

Depressive Disorder
- Does not meet the criteria for major depression and other disorders.

Depression in Older Adults
Clinical Manifestations
- Depressed, irritable, or anxious (may deny sad mood and complain of pain or somatic distress).
- Crying spells (or complaining of inability to cry or experience emotion).
- Unrelenting feeling of sadness.
- Indifference to others.

Associated Psychological Symptoms
- Loss of interest in usual activities, loss of attachments, social withdrawal, and reduction in gratification.
- Lack of self-confidence, low self-esteem, and self-reproach.
- Poor concentration and memory.
- Negative expectations, hopelessness, helplessness, and increased dependency.
- Recurrent thoughts of death.
- Suicidal thoughts.

Somatic Manifestations
- Anorexia, weight loss, pains, aches, and stomach problems.
- Insomnia, early morning awakening, or excessive sleeping.
- Psychomotor retardation.
- Feeling tired all of the time.

Psychotic Symptoms
- Delusions of worthlessness and sinfulness.
- Delusions of ill health.
- Delusions of poverty.
- Depressive hallucinations in the auditory, visual, and olfactory spheres.

Cognitive Symptoms
- Impaired concentration.
- Problems with memory.
- Indecisiveness.
- Recurrent thoughts of death and suicide.

Behavioral Symptoms
- Neglecting personal appearance.
- Withdrawing from others.
- Increased alcohol consumption or drug use.
- Agitation/anxiety.

Signs of Suicidal Intent
- Talking about death as a relief.
- Giving away possessions.
- Failing to take prescribed medications.
- Obtaining a weapon.

Nursing Interventions
- Assess client for signs and symptoms of depression.
- If client is depressed, ask if he or she has thought about committing suicide.
- Show interest and offer support; older adults may want to talk about their lives. Such "life review" talks can help older adults identify the main themes of their lives, express regret, and talk about their legacy.
- Avoid giving pat answers or advice.
- Identify the client's support among friends, family, and clergy.
- Remove implements or medications that can be used for suicide.
- Notify other staff, document your findings, and participate in the plan of care.

Bipolar Disorders
- **Bipolar I disorder:** Includes one or more manic or mixed episodes, usually with a major depressive episode.
- **Bipolar II disorder:** Includes one or two major depressive episodes and at least one hypomanic (less than full mania) episode.
- **Cyclothymic disorder:** Includes at least 2 years of hypomanic periods that do not meet the criteria for the other disorders.
- **Bipolar disorder:** Does not meet any of the other bipolar disorder criteria.

Client/Family Education
- Explain mood disorders in terms of their biochemical basis ("depression is an illness, not a weakness"), although often recurrent, chronic illnesses.
- Families and clients need to understand that early diagnosis and treatment are essential for effective management and improved outcome.
- As with any chronic illness, ongoing management, including pharmacologic treatment, is required.
- Reinforce the need to adhere to the dosing schedule as prescribed and not to make any unilateral decisions, including stopping, without conferring with health professional.
- There may be exacerbations from time to time, with a need to modify treatment. Help client and family identify early signs of regression, and advise to contact physician immediately.
- Work with client and family on side effect management.
- Address weight gain possibilities; monitor weight, body mass index, exercise, and food plans to prevent weight gain.

Personality Disorders

Cluster A Personality Disorders
- This cluster includes the distrustful, emotionally detached, eccentric personalities:
  - Paranoid personality disorder
  - Schizoid personality
  - Schizotypal personality disorder

Cluster B Personality Disorders
- This cluster includes those who have disregard for others, unstable and intense interpersonal relationships, excessive attention seeking, and entitlement issues with a lack of empathy for others:
  - Antisocial personality disorder
  - Borderline
  - Histrionic
  - Narcissistic personality disorder

- This cluster includes the avoider of social situations; the clinging, submissive personality; and the person preoccupied with details, rules, and order.
  - Avoidant personality
  - Dependent personality

Client/Family Education

- Educate client and family about the personality disorder. In this way, the client has a basis/framework in which to understand his or her recurrent patterns of behavior.
- Work with client and family in identifying most troublesome behaviors (temper tantrums), and work with client to develop alternative responses and anticipate triggers.
- For clients who act out using suicidal gestures, consider preparing an agreement that helps client work on impulse control.
- It is better to lead clients to a conclusion ("Can you see why your friend was angry?") rather than telling the client what he or she did, especially those clients with a borderline personality disorder.
- Because these are long-standing, fixed views of the world, they require time and patience and can be frustrating to treat.
- Although borderline personality disorder receives much attention, all clients with personality disorders suffer in relationships, occupations, and social situations.
- Client must be willing to change, and a therapeutic relationship is a prerequisite for anyone with a personality disorder to accept criticisms/frustrations. Some clients believe the problems rest with everyone but them.

Schizophrenia and Related Psychotic Disorders

Schizophrenia

- It is now accepted that this complex disorder is the result of neurobiological factors rather than some early psychological trauma.
- Onset is in the late teens to early 20s; it equally affects men and women.
- It is a devastating disease for both the client and family.
- It affects thoughts and emotions to the point that social and occupational functioning is impaired.

- About 9% to 13% of people with schizophrenia commit suicide.
- Early diagnosis and treatment are critical.

Types of Schizophrenia
- Paranoid.
- Disorganized.
- Catatonic.
- Undifferentiated.
- Residual types.

Signs and Symptoms
- The presence of two or more of the following for at least 1 month:
  - Delusions
  - Hallucinations
  - Disorganized speech
  - Disorganized behavior
  - Negative symptoms
  - Functional disturbances in school, work, self-care, personal relations
  - Continuation of disturbance for 6 months

Other Psychotic Disorders
- Schizophreniform disorder.
- Schizoaffective disorder.
- Delusional disorder.
- Brief psychotic disorder.
- Shared psychotic disorder.

Thought Disorders
- **Delusion of grandeur:** Exaggerated/unrealistic sense of importance, power, and identity.
- **Delusion of persecution:** Belief that others are out to harm or persecute him or her in some way.
- **Delusion of reference:** Belief that everything in the environment is somewhat related to the person.
- **Somatic delusion:** An unrealistic belief about the body.
- **Control delusion:** Belief that someone or something is controlling the person.

- **Circumstantiality**: Excessive and irrelevant detail in descriptions with the person eventually making his or her point.
- **Concrete thinking**: Inability to abstract and speaking in concrete, liberal terms.
- **Clang association**: Association of words by sounds rather than by meaning.
- **Loose association**: A loose connection between thoughts that is often unrelated.
- **Tangentiality**: Digressions in conversation from topic to topic, with the person never making his or her point.
- **Neologism**: Creation of a new word meaningful only to that person.
- **Word salad**: Combination of words that have no meaning or connection.

Client/Family Education

- Client and family need to be educated about the importance of taking antipsychotic medication to prevent relapse. Client will likely need medication indefinitely to prevent relapse and possible worsening of condition.
- Client needs both medication and family and community support.
- Once stabilized on medication, clients often stop taking their medication because they feel it is no longer necessary. It is important to stress the need for medication indefinitely and that maintenance medication is needed to prevent relapse.
- Clients may stop taking their medication because of untoward side effects. Engage the client in a discussion about medications, so that he or she has some control about options.
- Educate client/family that periodic lab tests will be needed.
- Some antipsychotics result in weight gain, so advise client to monitor food intake and provide dietary education as needed.
- Weighing weekly at first may identify a problem early on and allow for institution of a diet and exercise regimen.
- Early diagnosis, early treatment, and ongoing antipsychotic maintenance therapy, along with family support, are critical factors in slowing the progression of this disease.

Substance-Related Disorders

- Includes prescribed medications, alcohol, over-the-counter medications, caffeine, nicotine, steroids, illegal drugs, and others.
- Serve as central nervous system (CNS) stimulants, CNS depressants, or pain relievers.
- May alter both mood and behaviors.
- May be accepted by society when used in moderation but can be abused in some instances and illegal when sold on the street.
- Substance use becomes a problem when there is recurrent and persistent use despite social, work, and/or legal consequences and despite potential danger to self or others.

Alcohol and Drug Use Screening Tool
CAGE-AID QUESTIONNAIRE

1. Have you felt you ought to Cut down on your drinking or drug use?
2. Have people Annoyed you by criticizing your drinking or drug use?
3. Have you felt bad or Guilty about your drinking or drug use?
4. Have you ever had a drink or used drugs first thing in the morning to steady your nerves or to get rid of a hangover ("Eye-Opener")?

Yes to 1 or 2 questions = possible problem
Yes to 3 or 4 questions = probable problem
If CAGE-AID score >1 Brief intervention provided Yes No

RAFFT Questionnaire for Adolescents

- R: Do you drink to Relax, feel better about yourself or fit in?
- A: Do you ever drink/drug while you are by yourself, Alone?
- F: Do any of your closest Friends drink/drug?
- F: Does a close Family member have a problem with alcohol/drugs?
- T: Have you ever gotten into Trouble from drinking/drugging?

Two or more affirmative answers may indicate problematic substance use.

Substance Use Disorders

Substance Dependence
- Repeated use of drug despite substance-related cognitive, behavioral, and physiological problems.
- Possibly resulting in tolerance, withdrawal, and compulsive; involves a craving for the substance.
- Not applicable to caffeine.

Substance Abuse
- Recurrent and persistent maladaptive pattern of substance use with significant adverse consequences occurring repeatedly or persistently during the same 12-month period.
- Involving repeated work absences, arrests for driving under the influence (DUI), spousal arguments, and fights.

Substance-Induced Disorders

Substance Intoxication
- Recent overuse of a substance, such as alcohol, that results in a reversible, substance-specific syndrome (e.g., acute alcohol intoxication).
- Involves important behavioral and psychological changes (alcohol: slurring of speech, poor coordination, impaired memory, stupor or coma).
- Can happen with one-time use of substance.

Substance Withdrawal
- Symptoms that develop when a substance is discontinued after frequent substance use (anxiety, irritability, restlessness, insomnia, fatigue).
- Symptoms specific to the substance used.

Addiction, Withdrawal, and Tolerance

Addiction
- Repeated, compulsive use of a substance that continues despite negative consequences (e.g., physical, social, legal).

Physical Withdrawal/Withdrawal Syndrome
- Physiologic responses to the abrupt cessation or drastic reduction in a substance used (usually) for a prolonged period.
- Symptoms of withdrawal specific to the substance used.

Tolerance
- Increased amounts of a substance over time are needed to achieve the same effect as obtained previously with smaller doses/amounts.

Client/Family Education
- Denial is the usual defense mechanism manifested in clients with these disorders.
- When substance dependence/abuse is suspected, it is important to approach the client in a supportive and nonjudgmental manner. Focus on the consequences of continued substance use and abuse.
- Discuss the need for complete abstinence.
- Encourage family members to seek help through organizations such as Al-Anon, Nar-Anon, Alateen, and Adult Children of Alcoholics. These and other 12-step programs provide support to families dealing with the unique issues of each addiction.
- In some cases, medication may be required to manage the withdrawal phase. Benzodiazepines may be needed, including client detoxification. Cocaine abusers may be helped with desipramine, fluoxetine, or amantadine.
- Naltrexone, an opioid antagonist, reduces cravings by blocking opioid receptors in the brain and is used in heroin addiction and alcohol addiction (reduces cravings and number of drinking days).
- Educate clients and families about the possibility of comorbidities (e.g., bipolar disease) and the need to also treat these disorders.

Suicide

Risk Factors
- Mood disorders:
  - Depression
  - Bipolar disorder
- Substance abuse (dual diagnosis).
- Previous suicide attempt.
- Loss:
  - Marital partner
  - Partner
  - Close relationship
  - Job
  - Health

- Expressed hopelessness or helplessness (does not see a future).
- Impulsivity/aggressiveness.
- Family suicides; significant other or friend/peer suicide.
- Isolation (lives alone/few friends, support relationships).
- Stressful life event.
- Previous or current abuse (emotional/physical/sexual).
- Sexual identity crisis/conflict.
- Available lethal method (e.g., a gun).
- Legal issues/incarceration.

Suicide Interventions
- Effective assessment and knowledge of risk factors.
- Observation and safe environment (no "sharps").
- Psychopharmacology, especially the selective serotonin reuptake inhibitors (SSRIs) (children younger than 18 years taking SSRIs need to be closely monitored).
- Identification of triggers; educating client as to triggers to seek help early on.
- Substance abuse treatment; treatment of pain disorders.
- Psychotherapy/cognitive behavioral therapy/electroconvulsive therapy.
- Treatment of medical disorders (thyroid/cancer).
- Increased activity if able.
- Support network/family involvement.
- Involvement in outside activities to avoid isolation:
    - Join outside groups, bereavement groups, organizations.
    - Care for a pet.
- Client and family education.

Elder Suicide
Warning Signs
- Failed suicide attempt.
- Indirect clues:
    - Stockpiling medications
    - Purchasing a gun
    - Putting affairs in order
    - Making/changing a will
    - Donating body to science
    - Giving possessions/money away
    - Experiencing relationship, social downturns
    - Recent appointment with a physician

Situational Clues
- Recent move.
- Death of spouse, friend, or child.

Symptoms
- Depression.
- Insomnia.
- Agitation.
- Others.

Profile for Potential Elder Suicide
- Male.
- White.
- Divorced or widowed.
- Living alone, isolated, having moved recently.
- Unemployed, retired.
- Poor health, pain, multiple illnesses, terminal.
- Depressed, substance abuser, hopeless.
- Family history of suicide, depression, and/or substance abuse; harsh parenting; early trauma in childhood.
- Wishing to end hopeless, intolerable situation.
- Possessing lethal means (guns, stockpiled sedatives/hypnotics).
- Previous attempt.
- Not inclined to reach out; frequent somatic complaints.

Therapeutic Interventions

Anger Management

Early Signs of Anger (Preassaultive Tension State)
Muscular Tension
- Clenched fist.

Face
- Furled brow.
- Glaring eyes.
- Tense mouth.
- Clenched teeth.
- Flushed face.

Voice

■ Raised or lowered.

If anger is not identified and recognized at the preassaultive tension state, it can progress to aggressive behavior.

Signs of Anger Escalation
■ Verbal/physical threats.
■ Pacing/appearing agitated.
■ Throwing objects.
■ Appearing suspicious; expressing disproportionate anger.
■ Acts of violence/hitting.

Anger Management Techniques
■ Remain calm.
■ Help client recognize anger.
■ Find an outlet:
  ■ Verbal (talking)
  ■ Physical (exercise)
■ Help client to accept angry feelings and to understand it is not acceptable to act on them.
■ Do not touch an angry client.
■ Medication may be needed.
■ Speak in short command sentences.
■ Never allow yourself to be cornered with a client who is angry; always have an escape route (open door behind you).
■ Request assistance of other staff.
■ Medication may be needed; offer voluntarily first.
■ Restraints and/or seclusion may be needed.
■ Continue to assess/reassess (ongoing).
■ When client is stabilized, help him or her identify early signs/triggers of anger and alternatives to prevent future anger/escalation.

Behavior Therapy/Cognitive Therapy

Behavior Therapy
■ A form of psychotherapy; goal is to modify maladaptive behavior patterns by reinforcing adaptive behaviors.

Techniques for Behavior Therapy

- **Shaping:** Providing positive reinforcements at increasingly closer approximations to the desired outcome.
- **Modeling:** Learning new behaviors by imitating the behaviors of others.
- **Extinction:** The gradual disappearance of a response when positive reinforcement is withheld.
- **Time out:** Isolating an individual from the environment where the unacceptable behavior is being exhibited.
- **Systematic desensitization:** Helps individuals overcome fear of a phobic stimulus.

Cognitive Therapy

- A type of psychotherapy; focus of treatment is on modification of distorted thought processes and maladaptive behaviors.
- Used for depression; panic disorder; generalized anxiety disorder; social phobias; obsessive-compulsive disorders; post-traumatic stress disorders; eating disorders; substance abuse, etc.

Techniques for Cognitive Therapy

- **Recognizing and modifying automatic thoughts:** Recognizing negative automatic thoughts and generating positive alternatives.
- **Behavioral interventions:** Activity scheduling; graded task assignments; behavioral rehearsal; distraction.

Crisis Management

A crisis is a sudden event in one's life that disturbs homeostasis; usual coping mechanisms cannot resolve the problem.

Types of Crises

- **Class 1: dispositional crises:** Acute response to an external, situational stressor.
- **Class 2: crises of anticipated life transitions:** Lack of control over normal life-cycle transitions.
- **Class 3: crises resulting from traumatic stress:** Precipitated by unexpected external stressors; causes individual to feel overwhelmed and defeated.
- **Class 4: developmental crises:** Resulting from unresolved conflicts in one's life.

- **Class 5: psychopathological crises:** Precipitated by preexisting psychopathological illness, such as borderline personality, severe neuroses, or schizophrenia.
- **Class 6: psychiatric emergencies:** Situations in which individuals become severely impaired, incompetent, and unable to assume personal responsibilities; examples include individuals who are suicidal, drug overdoses, acute psychoses.

Four-Phase Technique of Crisis Intervention
- **Phase 1: data collection:**
  - Gather information regarding precipitating stressor.
  - Determine what prompted the individual to seek medical help.
- **Phase 2: planning of therapeutic interventions:**
  - Aid in the selection of appropriate nursing actions for the identified nursing diagnoses.
  - Consider the type of crisis, the individual's strengths, and available resources.
- **Phase 3: intervention:**
  - Use a reality-oriented approach; focus on the here and now.
  - Show unconditional acceptance, use active listening skills; attend to immediate needs.
  - Set firm limits on aggressive/destructive behaviors.
  - Assist the client in identifying the problem.
  - Acknowledge the client's feelings.
  - Guide the client through the problem-solving process.
- **Phase 4: evaluation of crisis resolution/anticipatory planning.**
  - Determine whether stated objectives were achieved.
  - Summarize what occurred during the intervention.
  - Review what was learned and anticipate how the client will react in the future.

Electroconvulsive Therapy

- The induction of a grand mal seizure through the application of electrical current to the brain.
- Used to treat major depression; mania; schizophrenia.
- Contraindicated with increased intracranial pressure and some cardiovascular diseases.
- Side effects: Mortality rate of 2 per 100,000; permanent memory loss; brain damage.

Milieu Therapy

Creating a scientifically structured, therapeutic community to affect behavioral changes and improve the psychological functioning of the individual.

Conditions That Promote a Therapeutic Milieu
- Basic physiological needs are fulfilled.
- Physical facilities are conducive to the goals of therapy.
- A democratic form of self-government is utilized; clients participate in decision-making.
- Responsibilities are assigned according to client ability.
- A structured program of social and work-related activities is scheduled as part of treatment.
- Community and family are included in the program of therapy to facilitate discharge from treatment.

Relationship Development

- The nurse–client relationship is the foundation on which psychiatric nursing is established; a relationship in which mutual learning occurs.

Essential Components of a Therapeutic Relationship
- **Rapport:** The primary task in relationship development; a sense of mutual acceptance, common interest, and trust.
- **Trust:** Confidence in the presence, reliability, integrity, veracity, and sincere desire of another.
- **Respect:** To believe in the dignity and worth of an individual regardless of his or her behavior; can be conveyed by calling the client by name, spending time with the client, being open and honest, and taking the client's ideas and opinions into consideration.
- **Genuineness:** The nurse's ability to be open, honest, and "real" when interacting with a client.
- **Empathy:** The ability to see beyond a client's outward behavior and understand the situation from the client's point of view; the ability to accurately comprehend and communicate the meaning and relevance of the client's thoughts and feelings.

- **Preinteraction phase:** preparing for the first encounter with the client.
  - Obtaining records.
  - Examining one's own feelings about working with a particular client.
- **Orientation phase:** becoming acquainted.
  - Creating a therapeutic environment.
  - Collecting data.
  - Setting goals; developing a plan of action.
- **Working phase:** accomplishing the therapeutic work to be done.
  - Maintaining trust and rapport.
  - Problem-solving.
- **Termination phase:** ending the therapeutic relationship.
  - Mutually agreed-upon goals have been met; client discharged.
  - Planning for continuity of client care.

Stress Management

The use of adaptive coping strategies in response to stressful situations.

Adaptive Strategies

- **Awareness:** becoming aware of the factors that create stress and the feelings associated with a stressful response.
- **Relaxation:** participating in activities that reduce stress, such as sports, yoga, breathing exercises, etc.
- **Meditation:** assuming a comfortable position, closing the eyes, casting off all thoughts, and focusing on one word, sound, or phrase; practiced 20 minutes once or twice daily.
- **Interpersonal communication:** talking out problems with a friend or therapist.
- **Problem-solving:** viewing the situation objectively and solving the problem using decision-making.
- **Pets:** studies show that caring for pets, especially cats or dogs, help pet owners cope with life stressors.

Maladaptive Strategies

- Smoking, drinking alcohol, using drugs, nail biting.

Defense Mechanisms

- **Compensation:** Process by which a person makes up for his or her perceived deficiency.
- **Conversion:** Expression of intrapsychic conflict through physical symptoms.
- **Denial:** Refusal to accept a painful reality, pretending as if it doesn't exist.
- **Displacement:** Directing anger toward someone or onto another, less threatening (safer) substitute.
- **Identification:** Taking on attributes and characteristics of someone admired.
- **Intellectualization:** Excessive focus on logic and reason to avoid the feelings associated with a situation.
- **Projection:** Attributing to others feelings unacceptable to self.
- **Rationalization:** Attempting to make excuses or formulate logical reasons.
- **Reaction formation:** Expressing an opposite feeling from what is actually felt and is considered undesirable.
- **Regression:** Retreating to an earlier stage of development.
- **Repression:** Involuntary exclusion of a painful thought, impulse, or memory.
- **Sublimation:** Redirecting unacceptable feelings or drives into an acceptable channel.
- **Suppression:** Voluntary and involuntary exclusion from conscious level of ideas and feelings.
- **Undoing:** Ritualistically negating or undoing intolerable feelings/thoughts.

Therapeutic Communication

Verbal and nonverbal techniques used to advance the promotion of healing and change; nonjudgmental; encourages exploration of feelings; discourages defensiveness; promotes trust.

Therapeutic Communication Techniques

- **Using silence:** Gives the client an opportunity to collect and organize thoughts.
- **Accepting:** Conveys an attitude of acceptance and regard. Example: "Yes, I understand what you are saying."

- **Using broad openings:** Allows the client to actively participate in the conversation. Example: "What would you like to talk about today?"
- **Restating:** Repeating the main idea of what the client has said; lets the client know whether or not he or she has been understood. Example: "So you are saying that you often become angry for no reason."
- **Reflecting:** Referring questions and feelings back to the client; a good technique to use when being asked for advice. Example: "What do you think *you* should do about your current situation?"
- **Exploring:** Delving deeper into a subject. Example: "Please tell me more about that incident."
- **Making observations:** Verbalizing what is observed or perceived. Example: "You seem tense today."
- **Presenting reality:** Defining reality or indicating one's perception of the situation. Example: "I understand that the voices seem real to you, but I do not hear any voices."

Therapeutic Groups

Functions of a Group
- **Socialization:** Allows social interaction with others.
- **Support:** Help from fellow group members in times of need.
- **Empowerment:** Bringing about improvement in existing conditions by providing support to individual members.
- **Informational:** Learning from other members of a group.
- **Task completion:** Assisting one another in endeavors that are beyond the capacity of one individual.

Types of Groups
- **Support:** Teach participants effective ways to deal with emotional, developmental, or situational crises.
- **Self-help:** Allow clients to talk about their fears and relieve feelings of isolation while receiving comfort or advice from group members.
- **Task:** Accomplish a specific task or function; focus is on problem-solving and decision-making.
- **Teaching:** Convey knowledge to individuals; participants also can learn from one another.

Laboratory Tests

Blood Testing

Color (Additive)		Color (Additive)	
Red (None [glass tubes] or clot activator [plastic tubes])		**Yellow** (SPS-sodium polyanethol-sulfonate)	
Red Marble Top or Gold (Clot activator and gel for serum separation)		**Yellow Marble Top or Orange** (Thrombin)	
Light Blue (Sodium citrate)		**Light Green** (Lithium heparin and gel for plasma separation)	
Green (Sodium heparin *or* lithium heparin)		**Pink** (EDTA)	
Lavender (EDTA–ethylenediamine tetraacetic acid)		**Tan** (Sodium heparin [glass tubes] EDTA [plastic])	
Gray (Potassium oxalater sodium flouride *or* sodium flouride)		**Royal Blue** (Clot activator [serum] *or* potassium EDTA)	

Note! For NCLEX Exam, Memorize Laboratory Values for the Following:

- Glucose
- Hematocrit (Hct)
- Hemoglobin (Hgb)
- Platelet count
- Potassium
- Red blood cell (RBC) count
- Sodium
- White blood cell (WBC) count
- Urinary specific gravity

(Source: NCSBN 2008 NCLEX-PN® Test Plan.)

Specimen Collection-Blood

General Guidelines
- Verify client allergies to latex, iodine, and/or adhesives.
- Never leave a tourniquet in place for longer than 1 minute.
- Avoid previous venipuncture sites for 24 to 48 hours.
- Never collect specimens above an IV site.

Procedure
- **Prepare the client:** Explain the procedure and offer reassurance.
- **Gather supplies:** Tourniquet, skin cleanser, sterile 2 × 2 gauze, evacuated collection tubes or syringes, needle and needle holder, and tape.
- **Position client:** Sitting or lying with arm extended and supported.
- **Tourniquet:** 3 to 4 inches above the intended venipuncture site.
- **Choose vein:** Most common and easily accessed are the median cubital, cephalic, and basilic veins located in the antecubital fossa anterior to the elbow. Veins of wrist, hand, or forearm also may be used but are smaller and more painful.
- **Cleanse the site:** Briefly remove tourniquet; cleanse site with an alcohol swab from the center out using a circular motion; allow site to air dry for 30 to 60 seconds. For blood alcohol level and blood culture specimens, use iodine instead of alcohol.

- **Perform venipuncture:** Reapply tourniquet; palpate vein with gloved finger; insert needle, bevel up, at a 15- to 30-degree angle using dominant hand; push evacuated collection tube completely into needle holder using nondominant hand or pull back syringe with slow, consistent tension.
- **Remove tourniquet:** If procedure will last more than 1 minute, remove tourniquet after blood begins to flow.
- **Remove needle:** Place sterile gauze over puncture site; remove needle; apply pressure.
- **Prepare specimen:** If using syringes, transfer specimen into proper tubes; mix additives with a gentle, rolling motion; label specimens with client name, ID number, date, time, and your initials.
- **Document.**

Arterial Blood Gases (Normal Adult Values)			
Tube/Heparinized Syringe		**Conventional**	**SI Units**
Green	pH	7.35–7.45	36–45 µmol/L
Green	PO_2	80–95 mm Hg	10.6–12.6 kPa
Green	PCO_2	35–45 mm Hg	4.66–5.98 kPa
Green	HCO_3	18–23 mEq/L	18–23 mmol/L
Green	Base excess	-2 to +3 mEq/L	-2 to +3 mmol/L
Green	CO_2	22–29 mEq/L	22–29 mmol/L
Green	SaO_2	95%–99%	95%–99%

Continued

Blood Chemistry (Normal Adult Values)

Tube	Lab	Conventional	SI Units
Red	Albumin	3.4-4.8 g/dL	34-48 g/L
Red	Aldolase	<74 U/L	<74 U/L
Red	Alkaline phosphatase	Male: 35-142 U/L Female: 24-125 U/L	35-142 U/L 24-125 U/L
Green	Ammonia	Male: 27-102 µg/L Female: 19-87 µg/L	19-73 µmol/L 14-62 µmol/L
Red	Amylase	8-16 mEq/L	8-16 mmol/L
Red	Anion gap	8-16 mEq/L	8-16 mEq/L
Red	AST, SGOT	Male: 19-48 U/L Female: 9-36 U/L	19-48 U/L 9-36 U/L
Red	Bilirubin, conjugated	<0.3 mg/dL	<5 µmol/L
Red	Bilirubin, total	0.3-1.2 mg/dL	5-21 µmol/L
Red	Calcium (Ca')	8.2-10.2 mg/dL	2.05-2.55 mmol/L
Red	Calcium, ionized	4.64-5.28 mg/dL	1.16-1.32 mmol/L
Green	Carbon dioxide (CO_2)	22-26 mEq/L	22-26 mmol/L
Red	Chloride (Cl)	97-107 mEq/L	97-107 mmol/L
Red	Cholesterol, HDL	>40 mg/dL	>0.9 mmol/L
Red	Cholesterol, LDL	<100 mg/dL	<2.59 mmol/L
Red	Cholesterol, Total	<200 mg/dL	<5.18 mmol/L
Blue	Copper	Male: 70-140 µg/dL Female: 80-155 µg/dL	11-22 µmol/L 12.6-24.3 µmol/L
Red	Cortisol	AM: 5-25 µg/dL PM: 3-16 µg/dL	138-690 nmol/L 83-442 nmol/L
Red	Creatine kinase (CK)	Male: 50-204 U/L Female: 36-160 U/L	50-204 U/L 36-160 U/L
Red	Creatinine	Male: 0.6-1.2 mg/dL Female: 0.5-1.1 mg/dL	53-106 µmol/L 44-97 µmol/L
Red	Ferritin	Male: 20-250 ng/dL Female: 12-263 ng/dL	20-250 µg/dL 12-263 µg/dL
Red	Folate	<2.5 ng/mL	<5.7 nmol/L
Red	Glucose	65-99 mg/dL	3.6-5.5 mmol/L

Blood Chemistry (Normal Adult Values)—cont'd

Tube	Lab	Conventional	SI Units
Red	Iron (Fe)	Male: 65–175 mcg/dL Female: 50–170 mcg/dL	11.6–31.3 µmol/L 9–30.4 µmol/L
Red	Iron-binding capacity, total (TIBC)	250–350 mcg/dL	45–63 µmol/L
Red	Lactate dehydrogenase (LDH)	90–176 U/L	90–176 U/L
Green	Lactic acid	3–23 mg/dL	0.3–2.6 mmol/L
Red	Lipase	3–73 U/L	3–73 U/L
Red	Magnesium (Mg^{++})	1.6–2.6 mg/dL	0.66–1.07 mmol/L
Red	Osmolality	250–900 mOsm/kg	250–900 mmol/kg
Red	Phosphorus	2.5–4.5 mg/dL	0.8–1.4 mmol/L
Red	!Potassium (K$^+$)	3.5–5.0 mEq/L	3.5–5.0 mmol/L
Red	Prealbumin	12–42 mg/dL	120–420 mg/L
Red	Prostate-specific antigen (PSA)	Male: <4 ng/mL Female: <0.5 ng/mL	<4 mcg/L <0.5 mcg/L
Red	Protein, total	6.0–8.0 g/dL	60–80 g/L
Red	!Sodium (Na$^+$)	135–145 mEq/L	135–145 mmol/L
Red	T3, free	260–480 pg/dL	4.0–7.4 pmol/L
Red	T4, free	0.8–1.5 ng/dL	10–19 pmol/L
Red	T4, total	Male: 4.6–10.5 mcg/dL Female: 5.5–11.0 mcg/dL	59–135 nmol/L 71–142 nmol/L
Red	Thyroglobulin	0–50 ng/mL	0–50 µg/L
Red	Thyroid stimulating hormone (TSH)	0.4–4.2 µIU/L	0.4–4.2 mIU/L
Red	Urea nitrogen (BUN)	8–21 mg/dL	2.9–7.5 mmol/L
Red	Triglycerides	40–150 mg/dL	0.4–1.5 g/L
Red	Uric acid	Male: 4.4–7.6 mg/dL Female: 2.3–6.6 mg/dL	0.25–0.48 mmol/L 0.21–0.43 mmol/L

! = **Memorize**

i = Memorize

Complete Blood Count (CBC) With Differential (Normal Adult Values)

Lab		Conventional	SI Units
Tube	Blood volume	8.5%–9.0% of body weight in kg	80–85 mL/kg
Lav	iRed blood cell (RBC)	Male: 4.71–5.14 × 10⁶ cells/mm³ Female: 4.20–4.87 × 10⁶ cells/mm³	Male: 4.71–5.14 × 10¹² cells/L Female: 4.20–4.87 × 10¹² cells/L
Lav	iHemoglobin (Hgb)	Male: 12.6–17.4 g/dL Female: 11.7–16.1 g/dL	132–173 mmol/L 117–161 mmol/L
Lav	iHematocrit (Hct)	Male: 45%–52% Female: 37%–48%	0.45–0.52 0.37–0.48
Lav	iLeukocytes (WBC)	4.5–11.0 × 10³/mm³	4.5–11.0 × 10⁹/L
	• Basophils.	0%–1%	0–0.1 × 10⁹/L
	• Eosinophils.	1%–4%	0.01–0.04 × 10⁹/L
	• Lymphocytes.	25%–40%	0.25–0.40 × 10⁹/L
	• β-lymphocytes	10%–20%	0.10–0.20 × 10⁹/L
	• T-lymphocytes	60%–80%	0.60–0.80 × 10⁹/L
	• Monocytes.	2%–8%	0.02–0.08 × 10⁹/L
	• Neutrophils.	54%–75%	0.54–0.75 × 10⁹/L
	• Bands	1%–3%	0.01–0.03 × 10⁹/L
	• Segments	25%–62%	0.25–0.62 × 10⁹/L
Lav	iPlatelets	150–450 × 10³/mm³	150–450 × 10⁹/L
Lav	Erythrocyte sedimentation rate (ESR)	Male: 0–15 mm/hour Female: 0–25 mm/hour	0–15 mm/hour 0–25 mm/hour

Coagulation Studies (Normal Adult Values)

Tube	Lab	Conventional	SI Units
Blue	ACT	90–130 seconds	90–130 seconds
Blue	Activated partial prothrombin time (aPTT)	25–39 seconds	25–39 seconds
Blue	Bleeding time	3–7 minutes	3–7 minutes
Blue	Fibrinogen	160–450 mg/dL	1.6–4.5 g/L
Blue	INR	Target therapeutic: <2	Target therapeutic: <2
Blue	Plasminogen	80%–120% of plasma	80%–120% of plasma
Blue	!Platelets	$150–450 \times 10^3/mm^3$	$150–450 \times 10^9/L$
Blue	Prothrombin time (PT)	10–13 seconds	10–13 seconds
Blue	Partial prothrombin Time (PTT)	30–45 seconds	30–45 seconds
Blue	Thrombin time	11–15 seconds	11–15 seconds

! = Memorize

Specimen Collection—Urine

Random
- Indicated for routine screening; may be collected at any time.
- Instruct client to void into specimen container.

Clean Catch (Midstream)
- Indicated for microbiological and cytological studies.
  - Males: wash hands; cleanse the meatus; pull back foreskin; void a small amount into toilet; void into specimen cup; secure lid tightly.
  - Females: wash hands; cleanse labia and meatus from front to back; void small amount into toilet while holding labia apart; void into specimen cup without interrupting flow; secure lid tightly.

Catheterized Random/Clean Catch
- Ensure tubing is empty and then clamp tube distal to the collection port for 15 minutes.
- Cleanse collection port with antiseptic swab and allow to air dry.
- Withdraw required amount of specimen using needle and syringe; unclamp tubing.
- Follow laboratory guidelines for handling.

First Morning
- Yields a very concentrated specimen for screening substances less detectable in a more dilute sample.
- Instruct client to void into specimen container on awakening.

Second Void
- Instruct client to drink a glass of water, wait 30 minutes, and then void into specimen container.

Timed (24-Hour Urine)
- Used to quantify substances in urine and to measure substances whose level of excretion varies over time.
- Collection should begin between 0600 and 0800 hours.
- Specimen container should be refrigerated or kept on ice for the entire collection period.
- The start time of the 24-hour collection begins with the collection and discarding of the first void.
- Instruct the client to discard the first void of the day and record the date and time on the collection container.
- Add each subsequent void to the container and instruct the client to void at the same time the next morning and add it to the container.
- This is the end of the 24-hour period.
- Record client name, date, and time; send specimen to lab.

Timed (24-Hour Urine)—Catheterized Client
- Follow same guidelines as with 24-hour urine, but start after the bag and tubing have been replaced. This is the start time and should be recorded on the collection container.
- Keep collection bag on ice or empty collection bag every 2 hours and add to refrigerated specimen container.
- Empty remaining urine into specimen container at the end of the 24-hour period. This is the end of the 24-hour collection period.
- Record client name, date, and time; send specimen to lab.

Urinalysis (Dipstick)	
pH	5.0–9.0
Protein	Less than 20 mg/dL
Glucose	Negative
Ketones	Negative
Hemoglobin	Negative
Bilirubin	Negative
Urobilinogen	Up to 1 mg/dL
Nitrite	Negative
Leukocyte esterase	Negative
Specific Gravity	!1.001–1.029

! = **Memorize**

Specimen Collection—Stool

General Guidelines
- Use standard precautions when obtaining/handling specimen.
- Use the freshest sample possible for best results.
- Specimens should not contact urine or toilet water.
- Preservatives are poisonous; avoid contact with skin.

Occult Blood (Hemoccult, Guaiac)
- Obtain collection card.
- Obtain a small amount of stool with wooden collection stick and apply onto area labeled "Box A."
- Use the other end of the wooden collection stick to obtain a second sample from a different area of the stool and apply it onto the area labeled "Box B."
- Close card; turn over; apply one drop of control solution to each box as indicated.
- A color change is positive, indicating that there is blood in the stool.
- **Note:** If client will be collecting specimen at home, instruct client to collect specified number of specimens, keep them at room temperature, and drop them off within the designated time period.
- Document results on client record and notify physician if indicated.

Cysts and Spores (Ova and Parasites)

- Open collection containers.
- Using the spoon attached to the cap, place bloody or white mucous areas of the stool into each container until preservative reaches fill line; do not overfill.
- Shake the container with preservative until specimen is mixed.
- Record client name, date, and time; send specimen to lab immediately after collection.
- **Note:** If client will be collecting specimen at home, instruct client to collect specified number of specimens, keep them at room temperature, and drop them off within the designated time period.
- Document specimen collection in medical record.

Specimen Collection—Throat Culture/Sputum

General Guidelines

- Use standard precautions when obtaining or handling specimen.
- Cultures should be obtained prior to the administration of antimicrobials.
- Document all specimen collections in the client's medical record.

Throat Culture

- **Contraindicated in clients with epiglottitis.**
- Instruct client to tilt head back and open mouth.
- Use tongue depressor to prevent contact with the tongue/uvula.
- Using a sterile culturette, swab both tonsillar pillars and the oropharynx; should elicit gag reflex.
- Place the culturette into its tube and squeeze the bottom to release the liquid transport medium.
- Ensure that the swab is immersed in the medium.
- Label specimen container and send to lab at room temperature.

Expectorated Specimens

- Instruct client to brush teeth or rinse mouth prior to specimen collection to avoid contamination with normal oral flora.
- Assist client to an upright position and provide an over-bed table.
- Instruct client to take two to three deep breaths and then cough deeply.
- Sputum should be expectorated directly into a sterile container.
- Label specimen container and send to lab at room temperature.

Aspiration/Biopsy

- **Aspiration:** The withdrawal of fluid that has collected abnormally or to obtain a specimen for diagnosis.
- **Biopsy:** The removal and examination of tissue; usually performed to diagnose disease or detect malignancy.
- Both are invasive and require strict sterile technique.

Bone Marrow Biopsy

- The aspiration of bone marrow from the sternum, iliac crests, anterior or posterior spines, or the proximal tibia in children.
- Used to detect specific diseases of the blood, such as pernicious anemia or leukemia.
- After injecting a local anesthetic, a small incision is made at the insertion site and a bone marrow needle with stylet is inserted into the red marrow of a spongy bone; may be painful.

Lumbar Puncture

- An invasive procedure in which cerebrospinal fluid is withdrawn through a needle inserted into the subarachnoid space between the 3rd and 4th lumbar vertebrae.
- Client is positioned laterally with the head bent toward the chest and the knees flexed onto the abdomen.
- Used to diagnose bacterial infections of the cerebrospinal fluid, which cause meningitis.

Thoracentesis

- Used to remove excess fluid or air from the pleural cavity to ease breathing.
- Needle is inserted below fluid level when fluid is to be removed; above fluid level when air is to be removed; chest x-ray is used to determine best site for needle injection.
- Client is positioned forward, leaning over a pillow or lying with one arm elevated and the other outstretched.

Chest X-Ray

- Chest radiography, commonly called chest x-ray, is the most frequently performed radiologic diagnostic study.
- Yields information about the pulmonary, cardiac, and skeletal systems.
- The lungs, filled with air, are easily penetrated by x-rays and appear black on chest images.
- A routine chest x-ray includes a posteroanterior (PA) projection, in which x-rays pass from back to front, and a left lateral projection.
- Aids in the diagnosis of diaphragmatic hernia; lung tumors; pulmonary disorders; cardiovascular disorders; skeletal disorders; and placement of endotracheal tubes, intravenous devices, nasogastric tubes, and pacemaker wires.

Colonoscopy/Sigmoidoscopy

- A procedure that enables a physician to evaluate the appearance of the inside of the sigmoid colon or colon by inserting a flexible tube into the anus and into the rectum and through the colon.
- The sigmoid colon or entire colon can be visualized either through the instrument or by viewing a TV monitor.
- Colonoscopy is considered the "gold standard" in the detection of colon cancer.
- Client's colon must be clean for the procedure to be complete and accurate; usually involves the client maintaining a clear liquid diet and drinking a colon cleansing solution, such as GoLytely® or magnesium citrate, the day before the exam.
- Most often used to detect and remove polyps or investigate the underlying cause of blood in the stool, abdominal pain, diarrhea, or change in bowel habits.

Computed Axial Tomography

- Commonly known by its abbreviated names, CT scan or CAT scan.
- An x-ray procedure that combines many x-ray images with the aid of a computer to generate cross-sectional views and, if needed, three-dimensional images of the internal organs and structures of the body.
- CT scans are performed to analyze the internal structures of various parts of the body. This includes the head; the spine; the chest; the

abdomen; and the reproductive organs where traumatic injuries, tumors, and infections can be identified.

■ The technique is painless and can provide extremely accurate images of body structures in addition to guiding the radiologist in performing biopsies of suspected cancers, removal of internal body fluids for various tests, and the draining of abscesses that are deep in the body.

Electrocardiogram (ECG)

■ A noninvasive test that is used to reflect underlying heart conditions by measuring the electrical activity of the heart.
■ Can be used to detect:
  ■ The underlying rate and rhythm mechanism of the heart.
  ■ The orientation of the heart in the chest cavity.
  ■ Evidence of increased thickness (hypertrophy) of the heart muscle.
  ■ Evidence of damage to parts of the heart muscle.
  ■ Evidence of impaired blood flow to the heart muscle.
  ■ Patterns of abnormal electric activity that may result in abnormal cardiac rhythm disturbances.
■ ECG leads are attached to three to five predefined positions on the front of the chest using a small amount of gel.

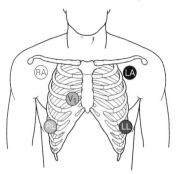

ECG Rhythms

Components of the PQRST

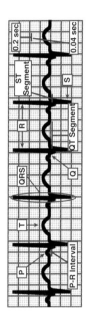

Normal Sinus Rhythm

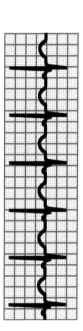

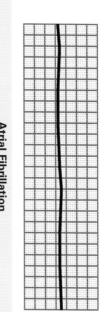

Atrial Fibrillation

Asystole

Atrial Flutter

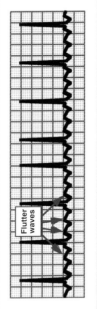

Flutter waves

Sinus Bradycardia

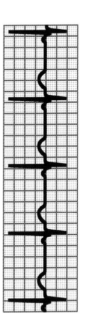

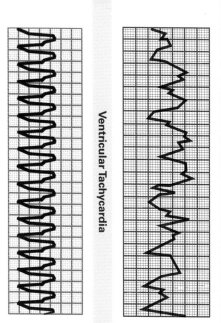

Ventricular Tachycardia

Ventricular Fibrillation

Magnetic Resonance Imaging (MRI Scan)

- A noninvasive, radiology technique that uses magnetism, radio waves, and a computer to produce images of body structures; an extremely accurate method of disease detection throughout the body.
- There is no exposure to radiation.
- The MRI scanner is a tube surrounded by a large circular magnet. The client is placed on a moveable bed that is placed into the magnet.
- The magnet creates a strong magnetic field that aligns the protons of hydrogen atoms, which then are exposed to a beam of radio waves spinning the protons of the body and producing a faint signal that is detected by the receiver portion of the MRI scanner. The receiver information is processed by a computer and an image is produced.
- For some procedures, contrast agents, such as gadolinium, are used to increase the accuracy of the images.
- Care must be taken to keep metal objects, such as oxygen tanks, out of the room where the MRI scanner is in use. The magnetic force of the scanner can cause such objects to become "projectiles," injuring those in the room.
- MRI is contraindicated in clients with artificial heart valves, metallic ear implants, bullet fragments, and chemotherapy or insulin pumps.

Positron Emission Tomography (PET Scan)

- A noninvasive radiologic study that involves the inhalation or injection of a radioactive isotope.
- Images are created as the radioisotope is distributed throughout the body; isotopes are absorbed by areas of increased metabolic activity, such as the rapidly dividing cells of a malignant neoplasm, which appear red or yellow.
- Allows study of various organ functions; may include evaluation of blood flow or tumor growth.
- Areas of low metabolic activity, such as in the brain of a client with Alzheimer's disease, appear blue.

Cultural Diversity in Health Care

Guidelines for Positive Cultural Interaction

- Assess the client's understanding of the English language and use an interpreter when needed.
- Identify who makes the decisions within the client's family (e.g., client, spouse, children, father, etc.).
- Ask the client how he or she would like to be addressed and by what name the client would like to be called.
- If unsure, ask the client about his or her culture and preferences with regard to nutrition, health care, visitors, etc.
- Be aware that culture greatly influences a client's interpretation of and response to health care.
- Be open-minded, accepting, and willing to learn.

African American Culture

Family Roles and Organization

- A high percentage of families are matriarchal and live below the poverty level; a single head of household is accepted without stigma.
- Grandmothers, aunts, and extended family members often provide assistance or take responsibility for children.
- Older people, especially grandmothers, are respected and play one of the most central roles in the family; **include grandmothers when providing support and health teaching.**
- Respect, obedience, conformity to parent-defined rules, and good behavior are stressed for children; most believe that firm parenting style, structure, and discipline are necessary to protect children from the dangers of the outside world.
- Churches play a major role in the development and survival of African Americans; most believe strongly in the use of prayer in all situations.

Communication

- Dominant language is English; informal language is known as Black English or Ebonics; **health care professionals must not stereotype African Americans as speaking only in Black English** because most are articulate and competent in the formal English language.

- Speech volume often is loud compared to other cultural groups; speech is dynamic and expressive and should not be interpreted as aggression.
- African Americans tend to be present oriented rather than past or future oriented.
- Greet clients formally by the last name, using the appropriate title until told to do otherwise; surname of the family is highly respected and connotes pride in the family heritage.

Health-Care Issues

- There is a general distrust and suspicion of health-care professionals; most seek medical care only when necessary; use of home remedies is common.
- Often seek clergy during illness; value prayer.
- Needed health care services may not be affordable for those in lower socioeconomic groups.
- ↑ Risk of keloid formation because of the tendency toward overgrowth of connective tissue; may lead to lymphoma and systemic lupus erythematosus.
- ↑ Risk of sickle cell anemia/disease, hypertension, stroke, chronic obstructive pulmonary disease (COPD), HIV/AIDS, cardiovascular disease, diabetes, misdiagnosis of psychiatric disorders, obesity, and lactose intolerance.
- Often distrustful of therapy and mental health services; may seek therapy because of child-focused concerns.
- Seek help and support through "the church," which provides a sense of belonging and community (e.g., social activities/choir); therapy is for "crazy people."
- Oral contraceptives are the most popular form of birth control.
- Postpartum period is greatly extended because of the belief that the mother is at greater risk than the baby; mother is cautioned to avoid cold air and encouraged to obtain adequate rest to restore body to normal.
- A bellyband or coin may be placed on top of an infant's umbilical area to prevent it from protruding outward; teach methods for keeping equipment and objects that are used on the umbilicus clean.

Diet and Nutrition

- Diets are frequently high in fat, cholesterol, and sodium and low in fiber, fruits, and vegetables.
- Food is used to celebrate special events and usually is offered to guests when they enter or leave a household.
- Being overweight is often seen as positive; it is important to have "meat on one's bones" to be able to afford weight loss in times of sickness.
- Foods such as milk, vegetables, and meat are considered "strength foods."
- Low levels of thiamine, riboflavin, vitamins A and C, and iron are associated with poor diet as a result of low socioeconomic status.

Pain Management

- Some perceive pain as a sign of illness or disease; regularly prescribed pain medication may not be taken if individual is not in pain.
- Some believe that suffering and pain are inevitable and must be endured; generally have a high tolerance to pain.

Death and Dying

- Common for burial service to be 5 to 7 days after death to allow relatives time to travel from far away to attend funeral services.
- Believe body must be kept intact after death; **explain legal requirements regarding autopsy.**
- Response to the death of a loved one may include sudden collapse ("falling out"), paralysis, inability to speak or see even though sight and hearing are intact; less likely to grieve in public.

Taboos

- Maintaining direct eye contact may be misinterpreted as aggressive behavior by some individuals.
- May not be accepting of same-sex relationships.

Native American Culture

Family Roles and Organization

- Most Native American tribes are matrilineal; land is not owned, but grazing rights are passed from mothers to daughters.
- Grandmothers and mothers are at the center of Navajo society, which is the largest tribe.

The relationship between siblings is often more important than the relationship between husband and wife.
- **When providing family care, no decision is made until the appropriate elderly woman (the gatekeeper) is present;** the gatekeeper should be located, otherwise time is lost.
- **A primary social premise is that no one has the right to speak for another;** thus children often are allowed to make their own decisions.

Communication
- Primary language varies from tribe to tribe; younger generations are bilingual (English and native language).
- Greetings should be formal.
- Long periods of silence are considered normal; loud talking is rude.
- Physical contact from strangers is unacceptable; shaking hands is okay.
- Respect personal space, which is usually greater than that of European Americans.

Health-Care Issues
- Extensive questioning during assessment may foster mistrust.
- Illness is unacceptable; older clients, even when seriously ill, must be encouraged to rest.
- ↑ Risk of alcoholism, tuberculosis, type II diabetes mellitus, pneumonia, influenza, gastrointestinal disease, and heart disease.
- Alcohol use is more prevalent than any other form of chemical abuse; related health problems include motor vehicle accidents, homicide, suicide, cirrhosis, domestic abuse, and fetal alcohol syndrome.
- **Check the immunization status of clients;** children are often not fully immunized because parents often have to travel great distances to seek medical care.
- It is often pointless to schedule appointments because of lack of transportation; must wait for others to transport them.

Diet and Nutrition
- Food has major significance beyond nutrition but is generally not associated with promoting health or illness.
- Corn is a staple; may be deficient in vitamin D because of high incidence of lactose intolerance.
- Sheep are a major source of meat; sheep brains are a delicacy.

Pain Management

- Most individuals are stoic and will not ask for pain medication.
- It is believed that pain should be endured.

Death and Dying

- Excessive displays of emotion are not considered acceptable among most tribes.
- Never suggest that the client is dying; to do so implies that the provider wishes the client dead.
- Organ donation and autopsy are unacceptable; body must go into the afterlife as whole as possible.

Taboos

- Direct eye contact or pointing the finger may be interpreted as disrespectful.
- Same-gender health-care providers should provide intimate care.

Arab Culture

Family Roles and Organization

- Muslim families have a strong patrilineal tradition; women are subordinate to men; young people are subordinate to older people.
- Older male figures assume the role of decision-maker.
- Children are dearly loved, indulged, and included in all family activities.
- Loyalty to one's family takes precedence over personal needs; sons are responsible for supporting elderly parents.

Communication

- Primary language is Arabic; speech may be loud and expressive and involve gesturing.
- Title is important; ask the client how he or she would like to be addressed.
- Shaking hands (right hand only) is acceptable; males should wait for females to initiate a handshake; etiquette requires shaking hands on arrival and departure.
- Good manners are important; inquire first about well-being and exchange pleasantries.

Health-Care Issues

- Same-gender health-care provider is strongly preferred.
- May be reluctant to share personal information with someone other than family or friends.
- Infectious diseases are common in newer immigrants; schistosomiasis infects about one-fifth of Egyptians and is Egypt's primary health problem.
- ↑ Risk of cancer, diabetes, hypertension, heart disease, sickle cell anemia, and thalassemia.
- Smoking and nonuse of seatbelts and helmets are major issues.
- Mental illness is perceived as resulting from witches or witching (placing a curse) on a person.
- In some tribes, mental illness may mean that the affected person has special powers.

Diet and Nutrition

- Pork, pork products, and alcohol are prohibited by Muslims.
- Medications should not contain alcohol.
- Bread should accompany all meals.
- Pass food to client only with the right hand.
- During Ramadan, fasting is required from sunrise to sunset.

Pain Management

- Pain medication is acceptable; most individuals are stoic around strangers.
- Take cues from family members regarding client discomfort.
- Closely assess the effectiveness of narcotics, such as codeine and morphine; some individuals have difficulty metabolizing debrisoquine, antiarrhythmics, antidepressants, beta blockers, neuroleptics, and opioids.

Death and Dying

- Clients should face Mecca (northeast from United States) when death is imminent.
- Autopsy, organ donation, and transplant are acceptable.

Taboos

- The left hand is used for toileting and is considered dirty.

Asian American Culture

- Refers to individuals of Chinese, Japanese, Korean, and Vietnamese heritage.

Family Roles and Organization
- Kinship traditionally organized around male lines; each family maintains recognized head of household who has great authority and assumes all major responsibilities of the family.
- Many Asian American families are transitioning from the extended family to the nuclear family unit and struggling to hold on to old ways while developing new skills.
- Children are highly valued; children born in Western countries tend to adopt Western culture easily, whereas their parents and grandparents maintain more traditional culture.
- Extended families are important; children may live with grandparents, aunts, or uncles.

Communication
- Primary language varies by country.
- Greetings should be formal.
- Direct eye contact may cause uneasiness in Chinese, Japanese, or Korean people.
- Touch Chinese, Japanese, and Vietnamese clients only when necessary.
- Shaking hands is acceptable when greeting Japanese or Korean people, but males should not initiate a handshake with a Vietnamese female.

Health-Care Issues
- Same-gender health-care providers are strongly preferred among Chinese, Korean, and Vietnamese clients.
- Assumption of the sick role is highly tolerated and long recuperation is encouraged (Japanese).
- May seek traditional or alternative treatments first before accepting Western medicine.
- Vietnamese are likely to refuse blood transfusions.
- Smoking and smoking-related illnesses, especially lung disease, are major concerns.

Risk of heart disease, cancer, stroke, pneumonia, asthma, hypertension, thalassemia, hepatitis B, and tuberculosis.

Asians tend to be more sensitive to the effects of some beta blockers, psychotropic drugs, and alcohol.

Diet and Nutrition

Rice is a staple in Japan, Korea, and Vietnam.

Tofu is a staple in China.

High intake of sweets may account for high incidence of tooth decay in Japan.

High incidence of lactose intolerance and iron-deficiency anemia.

Prefer beverages without ice in China.

Pain Management

May be reluctant to accept or request pain medication.

Death and Dying

Death is viewed as natural part of life cycle.

Responsibility for special arrangements is made by the eldest son in Japan and Korea.

Mourning may include offerings of food and money.

Vietnamese usually have a strong wish to die at home and are unlikely to consent to autopsy.

Organ donation and transplantation are acceptable in Japanese, Korean, and Vietnamese cultures.

Taboos

Open discussions about serious disease and death are unacceptable.

Direct eye contact may communicate disrespect to Chinese, Japanese, and Vietnamese individuals.

Pointing is considered rude to Vietnamese people.

Chopsticks stuck upright in food is considered bad luck to Chinese.

White and black are considered unlucky, whereas red is considered the luckiest color in Chinese culture.

Cuban Culture

Family Roles and Organization
- Traditional family culture is patriarchal, characterized by dominant, assertive male and passive, dependent female.
- Multigenerational households are common; the family is the most important source of emotional and physical support.
- According to U.S. standards, Cuban parents tend to pamper and over-protect their children.
- Honor is attained by fulfilling family obligations and treating others with respect.

Communication
- Primary language is Spanish; language is the greatest barrier to health care.
- Speech tends to be loud and fast by Western standards.
- Direct eye contact is acceptable during conversations.
- Greetings should be formal.
- Shaking hands and casual contact are acceptable, but necessity to touch private areas during physical exam should be explained.

Health-Care Issues
- May seek traditional or alternate treatments first; otherwise, Western medicine is openly accepted.
- Blood transfusion is generally accepted.
- Smoking and alcohol use are considered major problems.
- ↓ Risk of diabetes mellitus, obesity, and hypertension.
- ↑ Prevalence of tooth decay, gingival inflammations, and periodontitis as a result of high sugar diet.
- Cuban women have lower fertility rates than Hispanic women; attributed to the fact that women are in the workforce.
- It is essential to ask clients if they use folk practitioners; collaborating with folk practitioners may increase compliance with health prescriptions.

Diet and Nutrition
- Yams, yucca, plantains, and grains are diet staples.
- High incidence of lactose intolerance.
- Being overweight is seen as healthy, positive, and sexually attractive.

Pain Management

- Pain is expressed openly as verbal complaints; moaning and crying are not uncommon.
- Explaining that pain medications promote healing will help clients to accept pain medication more readily.

Death and Dying

- Dying persons are typically attended by large numbers of relatives and friends.
- Grieving is conducted openly, and mourning may be elaborate by Western standards.
- Candles are lit after death to illuminate the path to the afterlife.
- Organ donation, autopsy, and transplantation are generally acceptable.

Taboos

- Cutting an infant's hair or nails before age 3 months is believed to cause blindness and deafness.

Filipino Culture

Family Roles and Organization

- Although the father is considered the head of the household, the mother plays an equal role and most often makes decisions regarding health care, children, and finances.
- Parents and older siblings are involved in the care and discipline of younger siblings.
- Conditions such as mental illness, divorce, terminal illness, unwanted pregnancy, and HIV/AIDS are not readily shared with outsiders until trust is established.

Communication

- Primary language is Filipino; starting in the third grade, all children are taught English.
- Adults should be greeted formally.
- Prolonged eye contact should be avoided with a figure of authority or an older person; meanings are imbedded in nonverbal communication.
- Male health-care workers should avoid prolonged eye contact with females because it is interpreted as flirting.

Health-Care Issues
- High value is placed on personal cleanliness.
- May seek traditional or alternative treatment first; otherwise, Western medicine is openly accepted.
- Assumption of the sick role is highly tolerated, and family members readily care for the client.
- ↑ Risk of coronary artery disease, hypertension, type 2 diabetes, hypercholesterolemia, kidney stones, gout, and arthritis.
- Breast, cervical, prostate, thyroid, lung, and liver cancers are major threats to this population.
- Alcohol abuse and smoking are major problems.

Diet and Nutrition
- High incidence of lactose intolerance; milk is almost absent in the Filipino diet.
- Cold drinks, fruit juice, and tomatoes are avoided in the morning to prevent stomach upset.
- Daily consumption of garlic to combat hypertension is common.

Pain Management
- More stoic by Western standards.
- Pain medication may need to be encouraged.
- Most Filipinos do not seek care for illness until it is advanced, thus making pain management important.

Death and Dying
- Many are resistant to discussing advanced directives and living wills.
- Cremation is acceptable, but organ donation is not.
- A priority for the family is to gather around the dying person and to pray for the soul during the immediate period after death.
- Women generally show emotions openly by crying, fainting, or wailing; men are expected to be stoic and grieve silently.

Taboos
- Planning one's death is viewed as tempting fate.

Family Roles and Organization
- No institution in India is more important than the family; men exhibit superiority over women.
- The male head of the family is considered sacred by caste and religion.
- Parents strongly encourage scholastic achievement in children.
- Although parents accept the Westernization of their children, arranged marriages are still common.

Communication
- Languages fall into two main groups: Indo-Aryan, in the north, and Dravidian, in the south.
- Women often speak in a soft voice, whereas men tend to be intense and loud.
- Women are expected to strictly avoid direct eye contact with men.
- Punctuality and keeping scheduled appointments may not be considered important.

Health-Care Issues
- Heart disease tends to develop at a very early age.
- ↑ Risk of diabetes mellitus, hypertension, obesity, rheumatic heart disease, and sickle cell disease.
- Breast cancer is one of the leading causes of premature death in women.
- Dental caries and periodontal disease are prevalent.
- Alcoholism and smoking are significant health problems, especially among men.

Diet and Nutrition
- Vegetarianism is firmly rooted in this culture; some consider eating meat to be sacrilegious.
- Cereals supply 70% to 90% of total caloric requirements.
- Water is the beverage of choice with most meals.
- Women are not allowed to cook during their menstrual periods or have contact with other members of the family.

Pain Management
- More stoic by Western standards; self-control is valued.
- Women suppress their feelings and emotions during labor; **closely observe body posture, restlessness, and facial expression.**

Death and Dying

- A tenant of Hinduism is that the soul survives after death; death is a rebirth.
- Hindus prefer to die at home; the eldest son is responsible for funeral rites.
- A priest should be present at the time of death.
- The body is usually cremated and the ashes are sprinkled in the holy rivers.
- Women may respond to death with loud wailing, moaning, and beating their chest in front of the corpse.

Taboos

- Single-parent, blended, and communal families are not well accepted.
- Homosexuality may cause a social stigma.
- Avoid prolonged eye contact.

Mexican Culture

Family Roles and Organization

- Men are expected to provide financial support for the family, whereas women care for children and maintain the home.
- Some households are patriarchal, whereas others are matriarchal.
- Understanding the migration of family is important, including who has been left behind.
- The church is the *barrio* that often provides community support.

Communication

- Primary language is Spanish; emphasis is placed on verbal communication.
- Greetings should be formal.
- Shaking hands is acceptable, but physical contact during examination should be explained.

Health-Care Issues

- The family is considered a credible source of health-care information among Mexicans.
- *Curanderos* (folk healers) may be consulted for problems such as *mal de ojo* (evil eye) and *susto* (fright).

- Most migrant workers are not aware of the dangers of pesticides and herbicides because they are not used in Mexico; health education in this area should be a family affair.
- ↑ Risk of diabetes, diarrheal and parasitic diseases, and malaria.
- Sick role is highly tolerated; family members readily take on client's responsibilities.
- Blood transfusion is acceptable, but some may fear this because of the risk of HIV/AIDS.

Diet and Nutrition
- Almost all Mexicans use herbal medicines and teas; use of over-the-counter medications is common.
- Rice, beans, and tortillas are staples.
- Being overweight is seen as positive.

Pain Management
- Explaining that pain medications promote healing may help clients to accept pain medications more readily.

Death and Dying
- It is common to have many visitors when death is anticipated.
- Organ donation and transplantation are acceptable; cremation and autopsy are generally not acceptable.

Taboos
- Extraordinary means to preserve life are generally frowned upon.
- Older generations may regard direct eye contact as disrespectful.

Puerto Rican Culture

Family Roles and Organization
- Predominantly Catholic, most value the spirit and soul. Many believe in spirits that protect or harm and the value of incense and candles to ward off the "evil eye."
- Men demand respect and obedience from women and the family; women gain status as they become older for their wisdom.
- Children are the center of family life; male children are socialized to be powerful and strong and females are socialized to focus on the home and children.

Communication

- Primary language is Spanish and English; speech is fast by Western standards.
- Greetings should be formal.
- Shaking hands is encouraged; many enjoy sharing personal information and expect the same in return from health-care workers.
- Older women may require a larger personal space when interacting with men.

Health-Care Issues

- Women may need to consult husband prior to signing informed consent.
- Women have a high incidence of being overweight; diabetes is the third leading cause of death for Puerto Rican women.
- ↑ Risk of heart disease, hypertension, asthma, malignant neoplasm, unintentional injuries, and AIDS.
- ↓ Risk of lung, breast, ovarian cancers; ↑ risk of stomach, prostate, esophageal, pancreatic, and cervical cancers.
- Alcohol use and lack of condom use are significant risk factors.

Diet and Nutrition

- Most Puerto Ricans celebrate, mourn, and socialize around food; refusing food offerings may be interpreted as personal rejection.
- Rice and beans are staples.
- Being overweight is seen as a sign of health and wealth.

Pain Management

- Many tend to be outspoken when expressing pain.
- Pain medication is openly accepted.
- Older generations may not understand the concept of a pain scale.

Death and Dying

- Seek out the head of the family (usually the eldest son or daughter) for notification of a deceased client.
- Grieving may be loud and expressive by Western standards.
- Cremation is rarely practiced and autopsy is considered a violation of the body.
- Organ donation is regarded as highly positive.

- Open communication about physical ailments and sexuality is taboo.
- Never address client or family using terms such as "honey" or "sweetheart" because this is considered disrespectful.

Index

Page numbers followed by *f* indicate figures.